THE TANTRIC
SEX BOOK

THE TANTRIC
SEX BOOK

Cassandra Lorius

Thorsons

I'd like to thank Tantra teachers John Hawken, Leora Lightwoman, Hilary Spenceley and Charlotte Koelliker for their unstinting help and warm support.

Thorsons
An Imprint of HarperCollins*Publishers*
77– 85 Fulham Palace Road,
Hammersmith, London W6 8JB

The Thorsons website address is: www.thorsons.com

Published in the UK by Thorsons 1999
10 9 8 7 6 5 4 3 2 1

© Cassandra Lorius 1999

Cassandra Lorius asserts her moral right to be
identified as the author of this work.

A catalogue record for this book
is available from the British Library

ISBN 0 7225 3886 3

Printed and bound in Great Britain by
Woolnough Bookbinding Ltd, Irthlingborough

CONTENTS

FOREWORD

Essences of lily, lemon and lavender were wafted under my nose, and small segments of pineapple, figs and pomegranate teasingly popped into my mouth – all of which I savoured with a sensual pleasure enhanced by being blindfolded. Percussion instruments were gently rattled somewhere near my ears, and my skin was brushed with fabrics, feathers and fur. In this state of heightened sensitivity my hand was placed in the tentative clasp of my neighbour to explore. 'I don't know where this is leading,' I thought, 'but if this is Tantric foreplay, I want more!'

TANTRIC WORKSHOPS

Tantric workshops have had a bad press – often portrayed as excuses for orgies by the tabloids. Yet they're not solely about sex but sensuality in the broadest sense. SkyDancing's 'Taste of Tantra' workshops combine the Eastern practices of yoga and meditation with techniques from modern humanistic psychology, which focuses on developing the intimacy skills needed to effectively communicate and connect with our partners. Participants are led through a sequence of exercises designed to increase energy and sensual awareness, culminating in an 'Erotic massage' from your partner. Tantra involves letting the mind go and becoming more expressive through your body. Along with a sense of relaxation and playfulness comes a surge of energy, which you can use in creative ways to enhance your interaction with your partner.

Discovering Tantra was a revelation for me – not that it felt strange or exotic. It was more like coming home to myself. Feeling freely expressive, worshipping my own body, and being

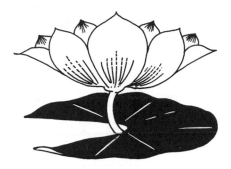

worshipped all felt natural and inevitable. Of course I am a goddess incarnate; I'd always known that – it was just that no-one else had!

My partner is also a natural Tantric; a very sensual man whose ability to love and connect continues to amaze me, in spite of other problems we have. Like all the men I've met on the Tantric path, he loves and honours women.

This honouring of women tends to run through the men who are attracted to, and stay on the Tantric path. They are usually more in touch with their feminine side, which makes it easier for women to express themselves more completely. Of course this doesn't mean that all relationship problems are automatically solved, but it's an important foundation for a couple who choose the Tantric path together.

Tantra means celebrating the love between you, and keeping it nourished and alive in a variety of ways, which this book will explore. It's all about being spontaneous and playing together, as well as nurturing a sense of your spiritual connection. Tantric practices are a way of finding or creating a path together that is filled with a sense of the sacred.

The key practice is to see your lover as truly divine.

When you accept that your lover is divine you can use the model of a divine relationship as an inspired template for your own. Even if you don't manage this challenging task you can experience a lot of joy and pleasure trying. And usually your sex-life improves greatly.

I was dissatisfied with my sex life before starting on the Tantra training. I felt that the full potential of my capacity for sexual pleasure had barely been explored, and that traditional sex therapy and self-help approaches had nothing to offer me. It wasn't that I had a sexual 'problem', or that I couldn't reach orgasm, but I felt a deep post-coital emptiness in spite of the love I felt for my partner. The models in our culture for a satisfying sexual relationship have more to do with ideas of stress-release and notching up orgasms than they do with our deepest desires for connection and intimacy. When I embarked on my first Tantra weekend workshop I had no idea that Tantric ideas and practices would resonate so strongly with me – it seemed like good fun at the time, and after several years of doing Egyptian dance, I wasn't shy about dancing and 'getting in touch with the sensual goddess within'.

But by the end of a weekend of ritual exercises, and yogic breathing with my partner I was on a literal high for the whole of the next week – it was so intense I wasn't sure I could put my serious hat back on and lecture abroad as I was scheduled to do.

As we drove back to London, through the spectacular fire-works of November 5th, I was filled with exuberance and an excitement with the discovery that getting in touch with my own passion could fire up my passion for life. My Tantric journey is not completed yet, and hopefully never will be. Working on a Tantric relationship, and incorporating Tantra into daily life are challenges that make life both more joyful, and more meaningful.

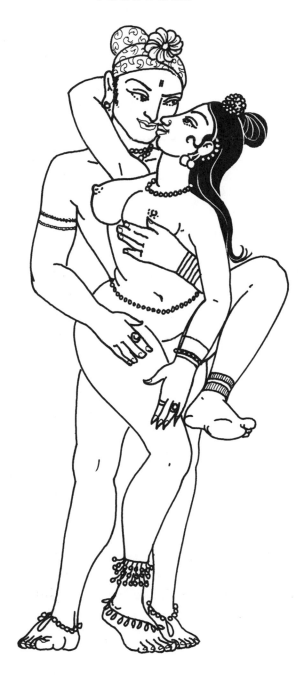

Part 1:
Introducing Tantra

'Bliss is my very nature
I need not do anything nor strive for anything to secure it.'

A Rishi's perspective translated by Deepak Chopra

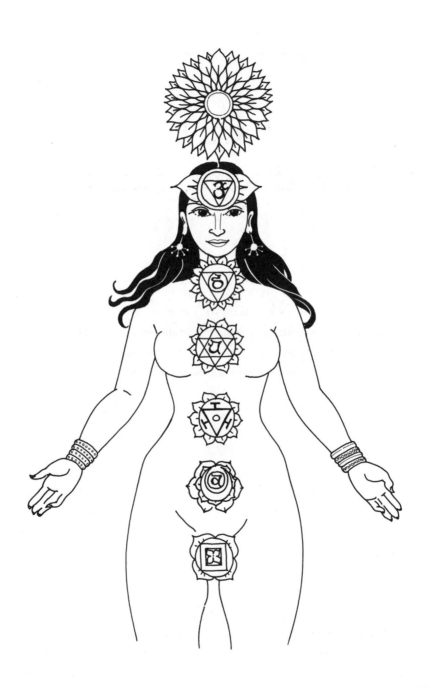

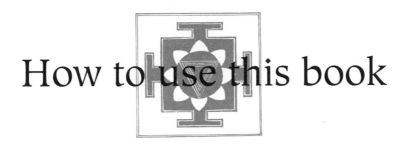

How to use this book

The first half of this book describes traditional Tantra as it has been practised by different groups in India over thousands of years. It looks at how Tantric teachings have been interpreted and how contemporary Tantra trainings in the West use some of these teachings. Contemporary trainings, such as the SkyDancing training I did, developed by Margo Anand in the US, are more properly neo-Tantra. They don't expect us to become familiar with the whole body of esoteric teachings of Tantra, but selectively take some of the practices and blend them with psychotherapeutic body work approaches to fit our current needs. In this sense, they can be considered a preparation for Tantra proper.

The book goes on to explore how the new forms of Tantra apply Tantric principles to contemporary life. I've quoted people who are on Tantra trainings to give you the flavour of what it means to real people, and how it influences the way they feel about themselves and their relationships. I've tried to weave a path between traditional Indian forms of Tantra, explaining some of the deep-rooted philosophy out of which these ideas and practices spring, and the ways in which Tantra can be applied to your life today.

The second half of the book provides you with meditations and exercises in the art of sexuality, which can enrich your relationship, and harmonize the energies between you and your partner. Use the structures and exercises suggested here to inspire you, change them to suit your own particular needs, and then let go of them. Otherwise the techniques themselves become just one more barrier to experiencing the flow of energy in all its power and simplicity.

The exercises may seem at times simple and at other times too complex, but if you enter into them with a spirit of adventure, accepting that whether you find them easy or difficult you will learn about yourself and your relationship, you will gain a lot.

If you get stuck, or find it difficult to create a safe space in which to do Tantric work, you may want to contact one of the many Tantra training courses available, which you can attend either as a single person, or in a couple. Check the resources section at the back of this book to find out about established trainings.

This book will enable you to taste what Tantra has to offer for you and your relationships, and gives you tools you can work with effectively on your own. The basic exercises can be used by single people, as well as couples. Although the exercises are geared towards heterosexual couples, they can be used just as easily by homosexual couples, since all couples can experiment with playing with the different masculine and feminine energies described by Tantra.

It doesn't matter if you're not interested in pursuing the philosophy behind Tantra, because these techniques will help you at whatever level you choose to take them on. If you just want to spice up your relationship, they will help you do that. If you want to follow Tantra as a spiritual path, this book will give you some insight into what that might involve, and encourage you to find your own personal teacher.

This book is also a very practical how-to manual, and regardless of whether you believe in any of the philosophical points of Tantra, these exercises will help you enter the realm of divine sex.

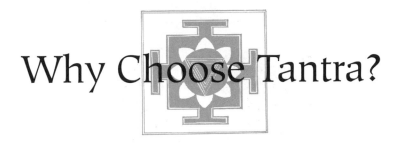

Why Choose Tantra?

Tantra is a path of sensual celebration as a spiritual discipline, which uses the erotic charge of sex to help us to connect with the divine. It is this openness to sexuality as a means of spiritual development that has led to Tantra's current popularity in the West – where we tend to focus on sex and self-development rather than the more radical message of transcendence.

The essence of Tantra is a relishing of earthly experience for the experience of divine bliss it can bring us. Sexual pleasure is used as a gateway to divine bliss, and sexual relationship is considered one of the fastest ways of reaching enlightenment. It's certainly the most enjoyable!

If your passion for life has been stifled within a stagnating relationship, an over-focus on mundane necessities or too much work, Tantra can help you to regain your zest for life, as well as take your relationship to new levels of love and connection. Tantra is a potent means of transforming your relationship – although, if your relationship has cracks in it, putting more energy into it will only expose the weaknesses! Tantra can make your relationship more alive and vibrant, more fun and sensual, and move you out of stagnation by showing you where and how to put energy in. The starting point of this process is to reaffirm the place of spirit in your life, and embrace spirituality in your sexual relationship.

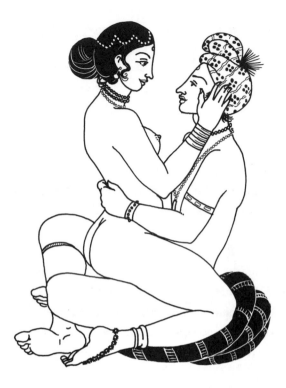

Essentially, Tantra encourages you to honour your relation-ship as a mirror of the divine relationship between Shakti and Shiva, the primordial couple in Hinduism, and to honour your partner as a mirror of yourself. Both you and your partner are divine, and seeing each other in this light helps you move out of petty squabbles and power struggles into affirming the funda-mental strength of your inter-connection.

Tantra sees your connection as a meeting of divine energies, rather than of two ego-bound psyches destined to act out past patterns and ways of relating that stem from your family back-ground. A psychotherapy-based way of looking at relationships can be of limited use, and Tantra replaces it with a more spiritual model. It teaches you how to unlock the energies within yourself and to use them to transform your experience of the world into one of bliss.

This involves becoming more aware of how your attitudes determine the way you experience your own reality, and how your level of awareness affects the quality of your relationships with others.

A strong sense of something missing is often what drives both women and men to explore other approaches to sexuality. The awareness of all the possibilities, all the different levels of experience we could have in love-making, and the knowledge that exquisite, divine sexual feelings are left untapped, are what brings us to Tantra. In orgasm we have a glimpse of eternity; letting go into something far bigger and more spacious than our orgasmic gratification. It's this experience of something vaster that keeps us fixated on sex, striving to repeat the experience. Tantra is the practice that allows you to attain that state without immediately losing it again. It allows you to maintain and extend it.

According to self-styled New Age guru, Barry Long, women and men are prevented from making love to our full potential, because we have not learnt how to make love with consciousness. Loving consciously involves Shiva (the man) receiving the divine energies of Shakti (the woman) in the act of love-making. Tantra teaches ways to make lovemaking more aware, and techniques for assimilating the energies of your partner in love-making.

Tantra has become increasingly popular in the Western world in recent years as we seek to address this underlying dissatisfaction with our intimate relationships, in spite of the hype about how much more sexual satisfaction we experience post the 60s sexual revolution. Survey after survey shows that we are not happier with our sex lives, nor our relationships, and Tantra offers us methods to work on these problems in a positive way.

Tantra workshops attract an equal number of men and women from a whole range of backgrounds. They tend to be in their thirties, forties and fifties, coming to Tantra as a result of the realization that the area of relationship, and sexual relating in particular, needs more attention.

Tantra is not a no-holds-barred excuse for sexual experimentation – it assumes that any work on sexual development is grounded in an egalitarian, committed and loving relationship. Within a relationship with a strong heart connection you can do the work of transforming sexuality into a more integrated way of being.

Tantra changes one's view of relationships. Couples become less dependent, jealous or neurotic. They tend to be more harmonious, fun and energy-filled. In the way of Tantra, you also discover that the relationship you seek outside is already within you. You simply need to learn about and cultivate the Tantric vision: a vital, bliss-filled approach to sex, love and life in general.

Sylvie, 50: I have to say no to casual sex now, even if I'm feeling turned on. I know that sex won't be satisfying because anyone who is not initiated into Tantra can't meet me at the level I can meet them. Every love-making is an experience of the sacred marriage for me – a deep connection of all the chakras. It helps for me to connect when I have my eyes open, when I can really look at my lover and be looked at.

When I experience love-making to that degree of merging I find it very difficult to separate afterwards. It's difficult to share these experiences with people who don't see love-making in this way. I call it paradise lost, when I'm aware of the many hours in my life when I feel unmet and as if I'm not connecting with people. Most of the time I have to sit in silence about my experience.

Tony 52: My sexuality has changed. I'm more relaxed and I have no sense of needing to achieve something. I'm not striving to make something happen anymore in my love-making. We've experimented with vetoing orgasms, both of ours and just mine. These days we have fewer orgasms, and we can stay in that feeling of excitement. Going to work with that feeling of excitement after love-making means that I feel alive. People at work comment on how good I look. I feel more open and that encourages others to be open. I find it easier to listen without being judgmental.

I also find I don't have to give advice — but if people do ask me my opinion, I'm more creative in thinking about solutions. I have more of a sense of humour, and generally have more fun. I can see the funny side of things as well as being serious — and that helps defuse situations I would have found embarrassing. This is my goal in working with Tantra over a period of time — to incorporate it more and more into my daily life. To have that sense of ease and flowingness in whatever I am doing. It's a combination of being more alive and full of energy, but being relaxed at the same time.

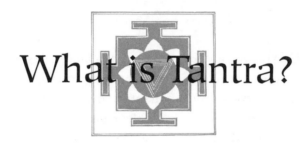

What is Tantra?

Tantra literally means a tool for expansion. In spite of the Eastern terminology, Tantra is an easy concept to grasp. At its heart is the knowledge that a powerful current of energy flows through us all, which needs to be harmonized.

The word *tan* translates as expansion and *tra* means tool. Tantras, the texts outlining Tantric practices, are literally tools for expansion. Tantra involves expansion on an energetic, psychological and physical level, and the teachings have been used for thousands of years as a tool to expand the boundaries of consciousness. Like all Hindu paths, it is primarily concerned with self-realization and enlightenment. Not through the usual route of suppressing desire and renouncing worldliness, but through harnessing the potency of desire, and pursuing bliss here and now. Tantra aims to harmonize life energies and resolve contradictions and conflicts in order to experience life as a flow of intense energy.

The word also connotes embracing. Tantra involves embracing all aspects of yourself. As long as you split off aspects of yourself that you don't like and hold them at a distance, you have no chance to integrate them and no chance of achieving wholeness. It is a heart-centred path, and invites its followers to embrace all of creation, in the name of love. You and your partner are both manifestations of love.

Tantra aims at total surrender – letting go of mental, emotional and cultural conditioning – so that universal life energy can flow through us as effortlessly as a stream. It's finding our way back to our existential roots, letting go into a sense of wonder and oneness with the universe, which spiritual teachers of all paths describe simply as love. On a more prosaic level, Tantric techniques aim to rekindle a lust for life through encouraging a more vibrant sense of self. Tantra is not a matter of rules and rituals: although it has its fair share of these, they are just structures to enable us to access what's really important – the direct experience of life.

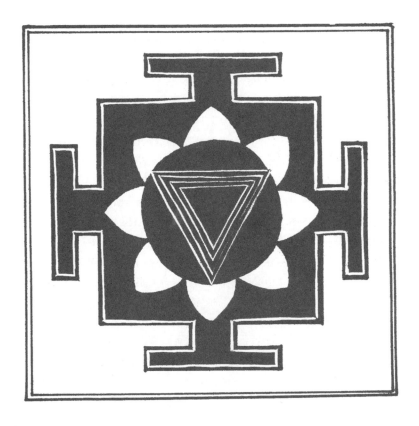

ROOTS OF TANTRA

The essence of Tantra is a non-hierarchical, non-judgmental, all-accepting approach toward experience. Tantra is an esoteric and magical tradition, which views everything that exists as part of the spiritual realm. In the words of the gnostic Hermes Trigemestus 'as above, so below'. The Tantric approach to the interconnectedness of everything is reflected in the saying 'everything is the essence of everything else'.

The roots of Tantra are somewhere in the pre-history of Indian religions: Hinduism, Buddhism and also Jainism. Tantric practices were drawn into a system around 1500 years ago, although its roots go back much further. It developed out of early matriarchal Indian culture, whose early goddess worship can be traced right through to today's popular Shakti cults. Different groups arose around different teachers, and cultivated their own practices.

Tantra is best understood as a group of texts and practices geared towards direct experience, rather than a spiritual system. The texts, called Tantras, outline methods for self-realization. Many of the Sanskrit texts take the form of question and answer dialogues between divine lovers, in which ritual practices and philosophy are discussed. Like all mystical paths that emphasize inner development, many Tantric teachings are esoteric – their spiritual meanings obscure to the uninitiated.

These methods were handed down orally, and practised by teachers and their followers. Tantra wasn't institutionalized, and there were no rules or hierarchies to limit access to the teachings. All that was required was the will to learn and the persistence needed to actually track down a teacher – since they didn't advertise themselves.

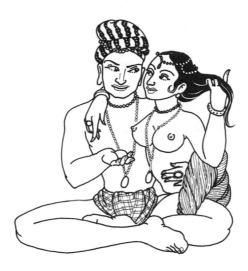

With the development of the Vedic system, based on a group of texts called the Vedas, introduced by Aryan invaders and subsequently favoured by Hindus, Tantric practitioners were marginalized. Asceticism, or physical renunciation, gradually gained ascendancy amongst Indians. The philosophy of learning through suffering, or working through suffering and hardship in this lifetime in order to earn future rewards in the next was regarded by Tantra teachers as a misapprehension of reality. Tantra says you don't need to suffer to attain enlightenment. Paradise is not in the next world, but here and now, if we can only see it.

Tantra developed partially in revolt against the proscriptive and caste-bound hierarchy of orthodox Hinduism. Some of the practices used by Tantrics were clearly conceived as blatant affronts to orthodox sensibilities. The central Tantric rite, called the five Ms, involved the use of five items considered taboo by Hindus. *Mady* (alcohol), *mamsa* (meat), *matsya* (fish), *mudra* (kidney beans – an aphrodisiac) and *maithuna* (ritual intercourse) are all used in Indian Tantric rituals as part of the core practice of invoking and identifying with divine Shakti energy. Tantric methods were concerned with challenging conventional taboos and restrictions – viewed as examples of limited, and limiting, thought patterns. Within Tantra, the process of achieving enlightenment was accelerated by confronting fixed ideas about caste, ritual cleanliness and gender. Taboos were broken as a way of developing non-judgement. These were ways of developing awareness that every experience, and every individual, was intrinsically pure. Rather than attempting to master the flesh by punishing it, or attempting to control sexual impulses through celibacy, sex and the body were used as a vehicle for spirituality.

Although the caste system has been in place for thousands of years in India, Tantra was always open to people of all castes. Tantric texts taught that all men and all women had equal capacities for enlightenment within themselves. In contrast to orthodox Hinduism, many early teachers were among the lower castes. Tantrics came from a wide range of backgrounds. Tantric meditations were designed to be adapted to any situation or occupation – a wine maker could distill bliss from the grapes of experience, while a weaver could weave passion using threads of freedom to produce a rug of enlightenment.

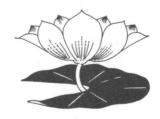

ACHIEVING BLISS

The goal of Tantra is to merge the phenomenal world with the divine, in one integrated, unified reality. Tantrics believe that in order to fully experience this reality all that is needed is a change of awareness. You are already divine, you just have to wake up to that fact. You don't need to change anything about yourself or work to achieve anything – you are innately divine.

Robin, 37: I thought it was normal to lose interest in sex as you got older. But I've discovered that my sexuality had just been put in a box to be brought out now and again. From childhood I'd been indoctrinated with the idea that sex is something good girls shouldn't do.

Now it feels like a natural part of life. I can experience things sexually and it doesn't have to involve sex. Sexual energy is just like any other quality produced by the different centres in the body – like the heart – but we don't allow the sexual feelings out. I realized it's always been part of me. If I hadn't learnt to hide it, it would be such a natural thing. Just to touch each other more. Sexual energy isn't just about sex – it's about aliveness.

On the workshop I got in touch with the more sensual side of sexuality – through touch and movement. We did some wild dancing, and afterwards standing still, someone touched me. Waves of intense sensation passed through my body. We don't know half of what we can experience, if we only just allowed ourselves.

Like all spiritual paths, Tantra is a philosophy with core values, which can be a problem for Westerners who are attracted to the open sexuality and the aura of permissiveness around Tantric practices. It is a spiritual path, which means that the search for bliss is not about pleasure for its own sake, since that is always transient and ultimately unsatisfying. It is about using worldly experience as a gateway to another perspective on our existence. A perspective that allows us to realize that we are already in a state of bliss – if we can only open ourselves up to that awareness. Paradise is here and now.

Unlike religions that separate existence into the earthly and the divine, Tantrics believe that our own reality is inseparable from the divine, and that you can't split them into two realms. Christian, Judaic, Islamic and Hindu traditions all split existence into a polarised duality of good and evil, heaven and hell, above and below. The path of Tantra is a direct path that cuts through dualism, not judging things as either good or bad.

We so often view our world as split into polar opposites, such as male/female, solar/lunar, heat/cold. Sexual union is considered to epitomize the essential unity of all things by the joining of male and female energies. Sexual ecstasy is the perfect example of the ways in which our experience of dualism can be transcended through experience – the experience of two bodies and souls merging into one.

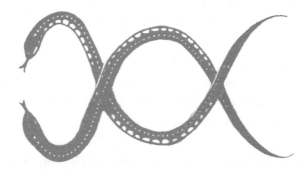

Catherine, 43: I no longer feel Tantra is something I need to do with my partner, or that it's just through sex. Ecstasy is very simple. It's not that intense, cathartic experience people think of, it's something very simple.

Ecstasy feels cool and still to me, and I can access it easily. I get into very ecstatic states through dancing, through pleasuring myself, or through simply looking at a flower. It's more a state of being. I feel it's about relaxing and opening up to that life force, that sexual energy.

It's a feeling of being at one with myself, and very much in my body. It's a sense of aliveness in my body. I can feel energy streaming inside me, little pulsations here and there. There's a warm feeling around my heart, a free and open feeling in my chest, and in my mind – the area around my third eye.

I find I'm accessing intuition more and more, and opening up to inspiration. There's a sense of unflappability, which comes from a deep sense of trust that I'll be able to deal with whatever comes my way. At the same time I'm much clearer about what I choose to do, how I choose to do it, and where I'm coming from in making that choice. I don't have to worry around in my head wondering what's right for me, I know it. Tantra has changed the way I am in life. I won't agree to do things that don't feel good anymore, whether in relation to work, or other people. I also just get on with what needs to be done – the boring, mundane things – without struggling against them.

Life isn't easier, but it's better. It feels richer, more meaningful, and I feel more in tune with myself. I feel heartful – more compassionate, but also more discriminating. There's a paradox between going with the flow, and somehow knowing that the flow is already chosen. All this is a conscious discipline. In every moment I can choose whether to deal with things in the old way, or with the consciousness I've developed through Tantra.

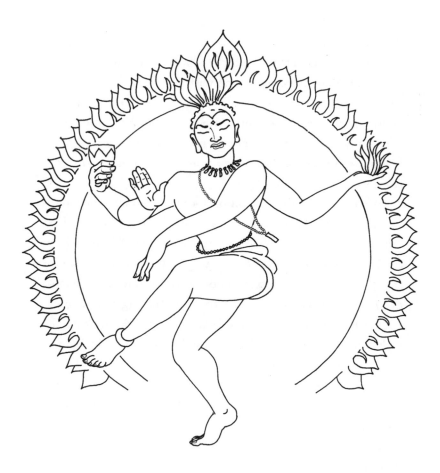

All humans are divine, and it is the discovery of and identification with the divine essence within that inspires seekers to follow the Tantric path.

SHAKTI –
THE FEMININE ENERGY

Hilary Spenceley, Tantra teacher: I love working with women, seeing the great healing that takes place with Tantra. I love seeing them step into their own unique beauty, which is totally independent of outside approval – that's what we call the place of the Goddess.

Tantra celebrates sexuality as a path to ecstasy. Tantric couples consciously honour the powerful sexual charge of the connection between them, which Tantrics consider to be a manifestation of the primal energy of the universe, called Shakti. Shakti is considered to be especially concentrated in a woman, and for this reason women are particularly venerated. Shakti, the energy of creation, and Kundalini, the individual powerhouse of energy that we all possess, are both thought of as feminine – and sometimes described as one and the same Shakti-Kundalini. Kundalini is also referred to as our inner woman, regardless of our actual gender. Each woman is honoured as an embodiment of divine Shakti, and each man recognizes and honours the feminine energies contained within him: the Kundalini. Tantra regards the powerful Shakti energy as innate. It's not something you need to build up or create, it's something you merely need to uncover in order to access.

Tantra's creation myth pictures the goddess Shakti making love with her consort Shiva. From this ecstatic union rains down a golden nectar which bathes the created world in bliss. Tantric writings describe the Hindu goddess Shakti as achieving seven peaks of ecstasy, each peak higher, stronger, and more powerful than the preceding one, until at the topmost she releases her nectar (female ejaculation). This nectar, amrita, is considered spiritual food for the universe, a pure joy, which radiates into the hearts of mortals.

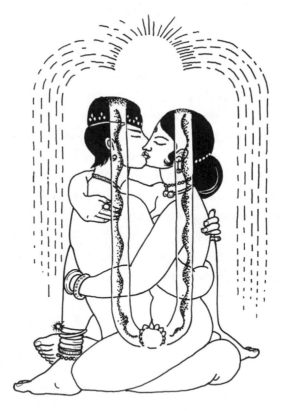

Divine couple in yab-yom. The image of divine love-making evokes associations of unity and complementarity; two interdependent aspects of existence.

The Tantric concept of oneness with the divine is often shown as Shakti-Shiva together in sexual ecstasy, a unification of both energy and consciousness. This image of divine unification is mirrored in what happens during mortal conception. During love-making a spark of bliss unites with the female and male generative fluids, and then creates a body in which to experience the true nature of reality – which is bliss. Bliss stays in the heart of each individual throughout life. In Tantra, this bliss is most easily realized through making love just as the original Shakti and Shiva did.

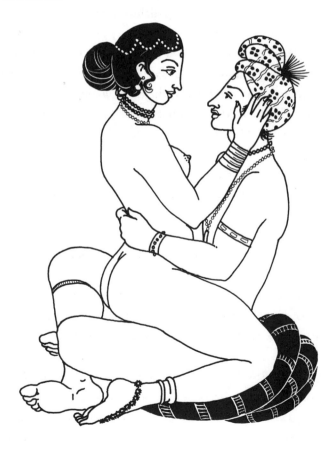

As part of the Tantric idea that God is in everything and everybody, you are encouraged to recognize the God and Goddess within yourself and your partner. In Tantra, this is the goddess Shakti and the god Shiva. Tantra also embraces the alchemical idea that each of us has an inner man and an inner woman, and that our sexual partners are external reflections of this inner marriage. When we unite with our partner, we unite with the other half of ourselves, becoming whole.

In fact, Shakti is not so much a goddess, as the creative force behind existence, who manifests in different forms. That's why she's not depicted as a single deity, but as a number of goddesses who represent the various qualities of this primal energy. So the wide range of local goddesses and gods revered by the Indians can be considered different aspects of primordial Shakti energy. Shakti is as changeable as the phenomenal world she has brought into being:

- As the divine seductress who initiated the act of love-making responsible for creation, Shakti is represented as Mohini – the temptress.

- As the maternal principle, Shakti is represented as Lakshmi, depicted holding a lotus flower, symbol of spiritual development.

- In her creative aspect, Shakti is depicted as Saraswati, who plays a musical instrument called the *vina*, and is regarded as the patron of the 64 arts one should cultivate in life – especially the arts of love.

- As in the cycle of birth, death and rebirth, all Shakti brings into existence returns to its original essence. In her destructive aspect she is depicted as Kali, the sabre-rattling goddess who wears a necklace of human skulls. She is depicted dancing on the corpse of her lover, the god Shiva. Shiva is often described as the footstool, or mattress of Kali – and if she's not dancing on him, she's mounting the erect phallus which is the only thing that animates his corpse.

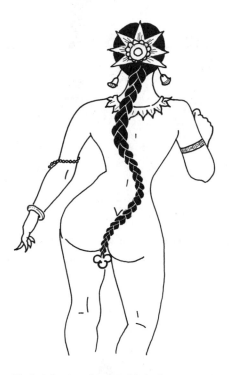

Shakti depicted as Mohini, the temptress.

Tantrics regard Shiva as a corpse without the energy of Shakti to bring him to life.

Shiva is the masculine equivalent of Shakti, the generic term for the male energy of consciousness, which needs Shakti to give him form. Shakti, the feminine creative energy is considered to be pure energy, and as pure energy is formless and flowing, she needs Shiva to give her consciousness. Each aspect complements and provides the identity for the other, as a means of becoming whole.

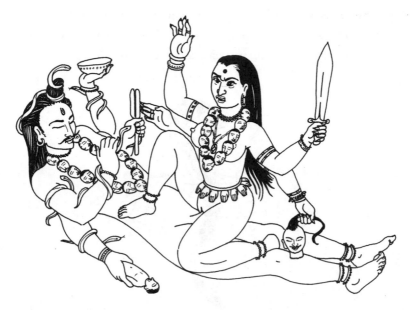

Shakti is often depicted dancing on her lover's chest, showing that she is the active principle without which Shiva would be nothing – quite literally a corpse.

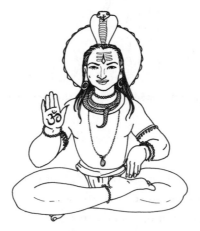

The kundalini energy is often depicted as a snake. In this popular image of Shiva, his personal kundalini energy has come to fruition at the crown of his head – the traditional site of his sexual union with Shakti.

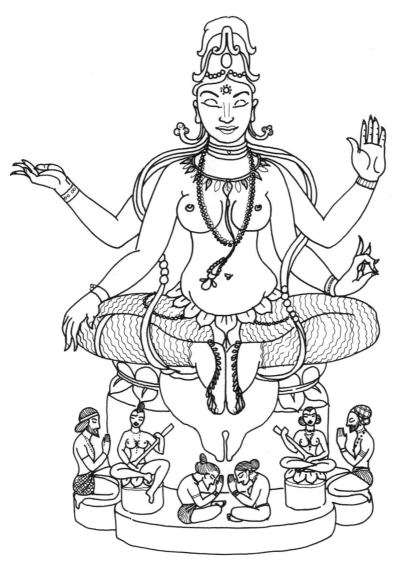

Shakti is considered to be especially concentrated in a woman, and for this reason women are particularly venerated. The sexual energy is also thought of as Shakti energy, in both women and men.

Tantra is unique in that it celebrates the power of sexuality, acknowledged in many cultures as the creative force behind existence. As a spiritual path it embodies a feminine awareness, since the divine principle underlying reality is feminine in nature. Just as all of reality is a manifestation of the divine, so too are women and men the embodiment of divinity. Men as well as women are honoured as god-like manifestations of the divine. Tantra advocates gaining knowledge of the divine through practical experience. Ritual sexual practices are considered the key to balancing the polarity in women and men, by unifying female and male energies in the body and aligning them with the cosmos.

SACRED SEX

Learning Tantra involves learning the art of spiritualizing sexuality.

Simon, 33: I've learnt to really slow down in sex. I can choose to go for it, or to make love another way. There's a choice about how to be. I spend hours making love, penetrating and then stopping to explore each other's bodies and cuddling and talking. Sex is no longer a one-off thing where you go for it and stop when you ejaculate. Now I can choose whether to ejaculate or not, now it's half and half. Tantric sex is more conscious. You're more conscious of what you're choosing to do, and conscious of exploring other things: exploring different feelings and physical sensations which you become aware of when you move away from bonking. For instance I hated being tickled, but now I love it.

John Hawken, Tantra teacher: In Tantric practice we learn to relax into excitement, especially with the pelvic floor muscle (love muscle or fire muscle) to allow the sexual excitement to spread, first of all from the genitals into the whole body, then beyond the limitations of the physical body into an expanded energy body, bringing us into connection and melting with our partner as the Other, and through them melting into the whole universe.

By consciously breathing the sexual energy into our higher energy centres, we can make love with our hearts and our spirits, celebrating sexual union as an all-embracing conscious experience of transcending aloneness into All-Oneness. On the level of pure energy, sexuality and spirituality become mutually completing aspects of our being.

Tantric practices involve a meeting on the sexual level. Sex is the beginning rather than the ultimate step in the journey you are taking together. Sexual practices are performed with consciousness of what you're doing, and why. More important than what you're doing is how you're doing it, and the intention you have when you're making love. Love-making with the intention of exploring real intimacy and connection with your beloved, and allowing yourself to see where that connection takes you, rather than limiting your focus to genital pleasure and orgasm, creates the right space.

Tantrics see sexual union as a means of achieving divine bliss. The pleasures of orgasm can be expanded into a whole body experience that links sex with your hearts and spirit. In developing the spiritual dimension of sex, you can enter the realm of divine ecstasy. You don't need to believe in Tantric philosophy, or follow its precepts to the letter, all that is needed is the right intention.

Tantra is not just about sex, it's about the free flow of energy within yourself, as well as with others. It's more about this flow of energy than about sexual intercourse or fancy postures for love-making. The emphasis in Tantric love-making is on non-doing – relaxing into pleasurable experiences and the energy connection you have with your beloved, rather than trying to build excitement and make something specific happen (orgasm).

You can use tried and tested Tantric techniques to help you

explore the connection between sex, heart and spirit. In 'Tantric sex', you focus on connecting genital sensations with the heart and the spirit, using breathing and meditation techniques, which connect up the energy centres in your body. Integrating the energy flow within yourself and with another expands your sexual experience. The exercises in the third and fourth part of this book lead to what SkyDancing teacher Margo Anand calls 'riding the wave of bliss' – divine sex.

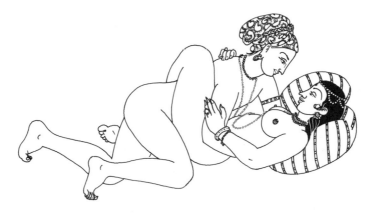

The following is a list of key basic elements that Tantric techniques use to help transform sex into an experience of the divine, which will be developed in Part 3:

• Foreplay starts before you even touch each other.

• The creation of a 'sacred space' using subdued lighting, candles and essential oils in burners, and a tray of sensual foods and drinks to feed your partner.

• The creation of a deep heart connection by spending a long time gazing at each other, feeling a sense of connection and harmony between you.

- The sharing of exercises to 'awaken the senses': feeding your lover titbits, wafting perfumes or essential oils under their nose, and stroking their skin with feathers or fabrics like fur.

- Tantra involves the whole body – so sex isn't just focused on your genitals.

- Focusing on the quality of sexual connection, not the quantity of sex.

- Taking time. Sex lasts much longer – instead of a few minutes the whole process lasts hours.

- Changing your orgasms from genital experiences to 'whole body' orgasms, where you feel energy rushing through your whole body.

- Breathing work: slowing down your breathing and harmonizing your breathing by breathing in and out together.

- Energizing the various energy centres in your body (see page 150), which is a practice of kundalini yoga, a type of Indian yoga.

- Imagining your breath is going right down to your pelvis, activating your sexual energy and building sexual fire. This is especially good for those who habitually suppress their sexual energy.

- Linking up the sexual energy in your pelvis, with your heart centre (over your heart) to get in touch with your loving feelings, and your third eye area (between brows) which is the energy centre (see page 151) related to your spiritual vision.

- Transcending the ego–bound aspects of your relationship, by focus-ing on what is essentially beautiful about the other person.

- Creating a convergence of breath and life-force through the subtle energy exchange taking place, in which the Shakti and Shiva principles unite within themselves and with each other.

According to Barry Long, on his *Making Love* tapes, the divine alchemy of sex cannot take place unless couples meet in deep love. If a man can open up to love and love his Shakti partner selflessly during love-making, he can express sufficient love in his body to reach the spiritual part of her.

This is how he can connect with the divine energies at her deepest centre. To be able to love woman this deeply is the masculinity man has lost. This is the conscious awareness, which Tantrics would call Shiva energy, that men have lost in this age of commitment phobia. To fully become an integrated man, a man has to be able to assimilate in his body the divine female energies a woman releases during love-making.

Woman cannot exchange her divine energies if neither she nor her lover is not yet integrated or fully aligned with love. The gap of unhappiness can only keep on growing.

Sex on the Tantric path is about exploring making love as the god and the goddess. You call them into your love-making and allow them to do with you as they will. It's about getting out of the way and allowing yourself to be surprised at what emerges, rather than trying to make something happen. Here, the physical activity is directed by the energy between you, so that love-making becomes a natural flow that is entirely unselfconscious and innocent.

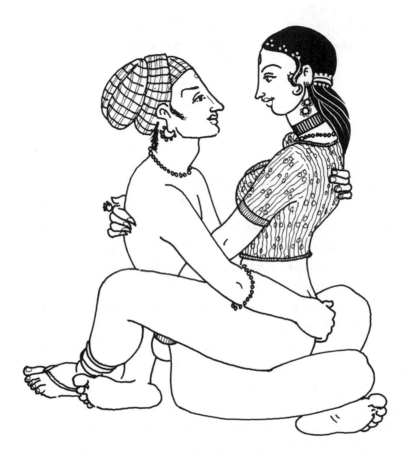

During ritual intercourse women are adored, the inner fire of kundalini is offered up, and the inner female and male principles are united.

THE TANTRIC ENERGY MAP

The key to understanding Tantra is understanding that we have a physical body and an energetic body. The energetic body is what animates our physical body, and permeates it. Sex is really an energetic meeting, a coming together of energy bodies as well as physical bodies. Tantrics visualize the powerhouse of our personal energy as a Kundalini snake, which lies coiled up in the base of the spine, waiting to be awakened and led up through the various energy centres in the body to the crown of the head. Preparation for Tantra involves focusing on this energy and drawing it up through the inner flute (central energy channel) in order to create powerful states of spiritual ecstasy.

Tantra doesn't assume that the subtle body exists in the same way as our physical body: it seeks to actively create the energy body through practices. It doesn't matter to the Tantric practitioner whether chakras, wheels of energy, actually exist or not, because in visualizing them, you are in a sense creating them. If

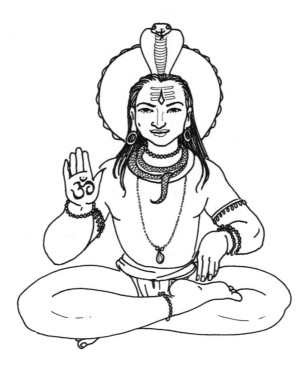

they help with the process of attaining a blissful state of consciousness, that's fine. Choosing to work with the energy body, as opposed to the more usual approach of experiencing sexuality as a purely physical activity, automatically allows you to transform physical experiences into spiritual reality.

CHAKRAS:
WHEELS OF LIFE FORCE

Mavis, 30: Nearly four years ago I had what I later realized was a Kundalini experience. It spontaneously happened during a Chi Gong class, with someone who was teaching us beginners very advanced stuff. I felt as if something was crushing down on my back, along my whole spine, and as if it was shaking me. My body was really hot one minute, then really cold. For three days I couldn't sleep, and after that I felt wonderful; I felt freed up, as if there were no boundaries between me and other people. I could look at people on the street and felt I could see into them, and I knew where their pain was. But it was very disorientating and everything felt blurred. My body and my mind were suddenly having to deal with a new reality, and these feelings kept coming back. I felt the Kundalini had opened me up, and there was no way of getting myself back together. The bodily sensations never stopped, but I can cope with them now, because Tantra has given me a framework for understanding them. Now I can see it's just energy moving in me.

It is considered dangerous to awaken the Kundalini energy without preparing and purifying the body. Tantra is a path of fire, and the power of the Kundalini energy when it awakens can burn us. Traditionally purification is achieved through a vegetarian diet, yoga postures and breathwork. These practices are then developed through the recitation of sacred sounds (mantras) and meditative visualization.

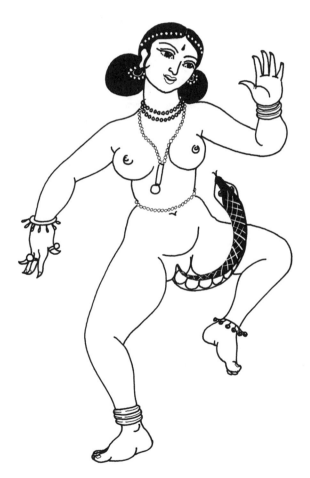

Kundalini snake energy emanating from the yoni.

Energy moving along the *sushumna*, the central energy channel of the body, is thought to pass through different energy centres or chakras (literally 'wheels' of energy), each of which have different associated qualities. The energy of the root chakra, at the base of the spine is described as solar energy and associated with the colour red, while the energy of that at the brow is lunar, and associated with the colour white. In fact, the energy of different chakras alternates between solar and lunar. Part of the art of drawing energy up through the central channel is to unite solar and lunar energetic qualities.

The energy body has been documented over thousands of years. In Tantric philosophy the seven layers of cosmic energy are reflected in the seven energy centres in the body – the chakras:

1 Nestled at the base of the spine is a golden egg. Inside this egg is the first chakra, the *muladhara*. The muladhara (root support) is particularly important because the creative force of the cosmos, the Kundalini, lies sleeping here. Visualized as a serpent, she sleeps with her body coiled into three and a half coils. In this chakra, you are working on the awakening of awareness, by awakening the sleeping kundalini energy.

2 The second chakra, found in the belly below the navel, is called *svadisthana*, (abode of the self), and is associated with creativity and the fertility of the great mother goddesses. It is associated with desire and sexual desire, as well as the tattva, or principle, of taste – both physical and preferential. As this chakra awakens, you are working on discrimination.

3 The third chakra is called *manipura*, (to shine like a jewel). It is associated with the element fire and is located in the solar plexus. It is

associated with the faculty of digestion, and in a broader sense, assimilation. In this chakra you are working on assimilation.

4 The fourth chakra, called *anahata* (without sound) is known as the heart chakra, because the heart rather than the head is considered the bridge between the body and consciousness. Energizing this centre leads to the harmonization of the other centres in the body. For this reason it is particularly important to awaken the heart. When the heart centre is awake it gives off a subtle vibration – the sound *om*, which is the sound of the creative energy of the void. In this chakra you are working on the ability to surrender.

5 In the throat region is the sixth chakra, called *vissudha* (purified), which is connected with the feminine power of creation. Known as the throat centre, it is connected with sound (mantras) and hearing, speech and silence, inhaling and exhaling, and the divine metabolism of Shiva and Shakti. This is the chakra in which you work on balance.

6 The brow centre is called *ajna* (command from above), and is represented by two lotus petals connected to a lunar disc, which is positioned to receive the nectar that drips down from the thousand-petal lotus at the crown of the head. It is thought to be the bridge between our higher mind and lower mind. It is the meeting place of the three main energetic channels, and is connected to the life-force. Situated in what we call the third eye, at the root of the nose, it has the function of psychic vision, or clairvoyance.

7 The crown centre is the seventh chakra, called the *sahasrara*, (thousand-spoked), and is located over the fontanel. It is usually depicted as a thousand-petal lotus, representing the full flowering of the subtle body into enlightenment. Tantric practitioners see this as the seat of

the divine couple Shakti and Shiva, whose unification brings about a state of bliss and enlightenment.

Tantra conceptualizes personal Shakti power, or Kundalini, as lying latent at the base of the spine until activated byTantric practices, when she arises up into the crown chakra and unites with Shiva.

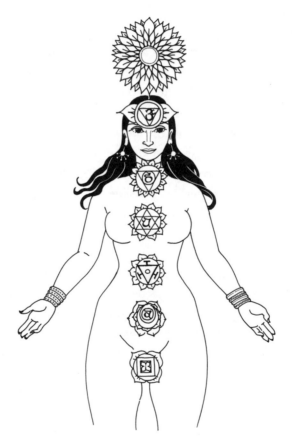

The energy body has been documented over thousands of years. The body's energy system is considered a microcosm of the macrocosm, which is the universe. In Tantric philosophy the seven layers of cosmic energy are reflected in the seven energy centres in the body – the chakras.

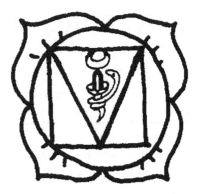

The symbol for the first chakra is a square (standing for the element earth) enclosed by four fiery red petals, inside which is a downward pointing triangle (symbolizing the vulva or yoni, the primordial fount of creation). Inside the yoni is a yoni-lingam (vulva and penis), around which the Kundalini snake is coiled, and which is covered by the crescent moon, (symbol of the divine source of all energy).

Yogis hold that the flow of energy upwards is blocked in a person in whom the Kundalini energy is still sleeping. The aim of Tantric yoga practices is to awaken this Kundalini-Shakti energy and to move it through the energetic blocks within the chakra system.

> ***John Hawken, Tantra teacher***: Tantra is about empowering yourself by rejecting external systems of ideas which tell you how you should be opening the heart. The key to real wisdom lies in your heart already. You are always in contact and in harmony with the whole – Tantra is about waking up to that knowledge. It doesn't happen through the mind, but by building up your energy and opening the chakras.

TANTRIC PRACTICES

Pip, 46: I was in a stone circle with my partner. We were lying under the central stone, dozing into the energies. Everything outside the circle disappeared. We felt both connected and independent at the same time, and I was waiting with a sense of expectancy. The energy felt very high and I tried to see what would unfold by relaxing into what was already there.

I asked my partner to lie on her front, and found myself tracing quite specific designs on her back. Lines up her back which spiralled into her shoulder blades and back down again three times on each side. The thought came to me that I was unfurling the wings of an angel, and allowing energy to open up. She began to dance tentatively, exploring this fine feeling. She looked like an elf or a fairy, both innocent and raunchy, as she danced around barefoot and topless. In her dance she'd become an energy being. Then she climbed up the central stone, which leans like a giant phallus, and perched onto the tip, looking like an amazing 'playboy of the year' image.

I felt it was a taste of how it is to touch paradise while still being on earth. That's how we want to live our life together.

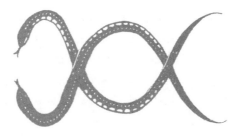

Tantra is not particularly concerned with dry philosophical spec-ulation, and the texts have little to add to Hindu or Buddhist phi-losophy, except for their emphasis on lived experience. Tantras are not concerned with splitting hairs about how to define the absolute: Tantric practices are geared towards creating a different subjectivity from the one we're used to, a different way of experi-encing ourselves and the world. The techniques can seem elabo-rate to us, because they're not part of our own background cultural knowledge. They've been refined over thousands of years, and are firmly embedded in a particular Hindu way of looking at reality, yet in spite of this they're simple and accessible. It's not necessary for modern Western practitioners to learn all the subtleties of the complex body maps and cosmologies familiar to Eastern Tantric practitioners. What's most important is devel-oping a heart-centred *modus operandi*, and using some sort of med-itation practice to experience these feelings of non-duality.

In meditation it is particularly important to focus on the heart area. Once this energy centre has been balanced, it will tend to harmonize the others automati-cally. A simple visualization for cleansing the heart chakra is to imagine your body wrapped in a ball of golden light, like a cocoon. Then, imagine a clear emer-ald green light in the heart area of your chest, which gradually permeates your whole body, and expands to colour the golden ball a bright emerald green. You can do this meditation with your partner as well, visualizing the cocoon around both your bodies.

Traditional Tantric practices involve purifying the body for Tantra through a vegetarian diet and through breathing tech-niques (known as pranayama), and working on the body's flexi-bility through the physical postures of hatha yoga. Then the work of awakening and raising the Kundalini-Shakti energy through the chakras can begin. Kundalini yoga uses a range of techniques to harness the libidinal energy of the body for spiritual development, including visualizations, breathing, sound (mantra) and gestures (mudras). In order to work with the energy body, meditation and visualizations are used to influence the body's subtle physiology as well as to deepen experience.

A traditional Tantric ritual involved investing space with sacredness through rituals: for instance, drawing the fundamental triangle mandala shape (yantra) on the ground facing north, or internally visualizing a yantra and the associated deity. Then the yogi recited lots of mantras to worship, invoke and identify with particular deities. Ritual food and drink were taken, and sometimes hemp, before finally making love while using visualizations to sanctify the ritual.

Maithuna is the traditional ritual practice of making love as the divine, recreating the moment of creation as Shakti and Shiva.

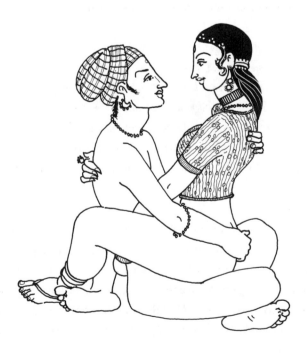

SACRED TOOLS: MANTRAS AND YANTRAS

Mantras are sacred sounds chanted by the adept to bring them into alignment with the energies of the cosmos. The famous mantra *om* is considered to be the sound of the universe humming. It is only when we have cleared our subtle body enough, and are able to enter states of deep meditation, that we can hear this spontaneous vibration of the universe, which is always resonating with energy.

Mantras – words of power

Seed syllables, which create the appropriate spiritual intention:

Aim	seed syllable identifying self with teacher
Hrim	seed syllable of shakti
Klim	seed of desire
Krim	seed of union
Shrim	seed of delight
Trim	seed of fire
Strim	seed of peace
Hlim	seed of protection

Another series of sacred sounds, associated with the chakras:

Lam	base chakra (muladhara)
Vam	sacrum (svadhisthana)
Ram	solar plexus (manipura)
Yam	heart chakra (anahata)

| Ham | throat chakra (vissudha) |
| Om | brow chakra (ajna) |

Mandala is Sanskrit for circle. It describes the outdoor earthen platform used for rituals, as well as being a generic term for a ritual space, and a gathering of yogis. Mandala also refers to the yoni in Tantric usage, which means an enclosed sacred space as well as the female genitals.

Mandalas are used for the ritual in which a spiritual teacher assigns a mantra (sacred sound) to her or his student. Traditionally, the teacher designs a mandala with four gates in each direction, made with coloured powders. The teacher invests the mandala with sacred power through purification practices, mantra recitation, and the visualization of deities inside the mandala. Within this space the student receives his spiritual instruction about which mantras to use for invoking deities. Traditionally, the reciting of mantras is thought to be worthless without having had some sort of initiation ritual to empower the power word.

Yantras are more simple geometric designs, which represent the energies of a particular deity. They are drawn out on the ground in sand or flour, or drawn on paper or wood, or engraved into metal. Geometric symbols such as squares or triangles are drawn within four gates surrounded by a circle of lotus petals. The dot in the centre is called a *bindu*, or energy spot. It represents the matrix of creation, which is the source of the yantra's power.

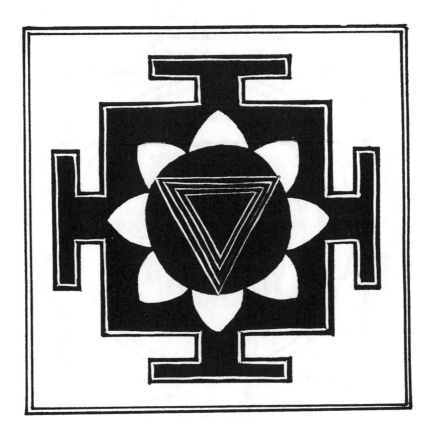

Yantras and mandalas are visual representations of inner and outer energy processes in geometric form. They are used in meditation to help the meditator align themselves with appropriate energy flows.

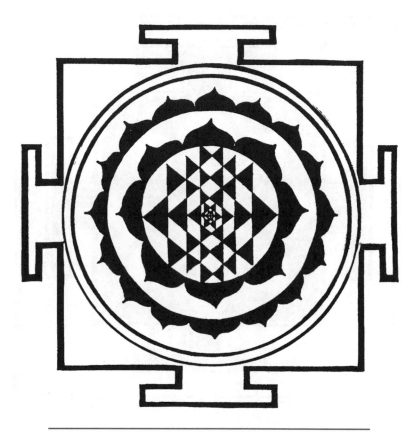

The famous shri yantra, used on the cover of this book, is dedicated to a form of the goddess, Tripura Sundari. The design is made of five downward pointing triangles, which represent Shakti energy, and four upward pointing triangles, which symbolize Shiva energy. Where they intersect they form 43 small triangles, or yonis. This is encircled by 29 mother deities, then another sixteen. Another circle of 16 lunar energies surrounds these, then sixteen lotus petals, symbol of transformation, containing more deities. The central energy point or bindu, represents Shakti power, which is the locus of bliss.

Ritual sexual postures are also called *yantras,* because they create an energy field through the different energy centres in the body. They unite the energy centres of one body with the energy centres of the partner.

Mudra usually refers to a ritual gesture: a gesture using the hands which invokes the presence of a deity. It also refers to the toasted kidney beans that are used as an aphrodisiac in Tantric rituals, and in Tantric Buddhism actually refers to the female partner in couple rituals (maithuna).

Mudras are thought of as seals. They help the practitioner identify with the deity and then seal those energies in the body. The 'yoni-mudra' is a classic gesture for the goddess, in which the fingers are interlaced with each other. There are seals for producing *amrita*, the ambrosial nectar of bliss, and others for enhancing meditation states. For instance, the 'seal of wisdom' is used while sitting in the 'lotus' or 'hero' posture for meditation, to focus and concentrate meditation.

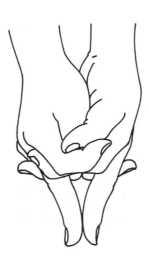

SEXUAL ICONS

Daniel Odier (author of Tantric Quest): The phallus of
Shiva is erect because it is raised to full consciousness, and
in full consciousness it penetrates the universe. The vulva
of Shakti is open because in full consciousness she lets the
universe penetrate her ... At the core of their mutual penetration supreme consciousness reigns.

Graphic images and sculptured representations of genitals are
worshipped as symbols for the female and male energies that
together make up existence.

Yoni is a sanskrit word for the vagina that connotes sacred
space or sanctum. In Tantra, the yoni is worshipped with love
and respect, as the gateway to a direct experience of the divine, as
well as the source of universal bliss. Yoni essence is drunk by
Tantrics. At a famous temple in Assam, where in one myth the
goddess's yoni fell to earth, spring water comes through a cleft in
the rock. In summer, red oxide colours the water red, and this
water is drunk in honour of the menstruation of the goddess.

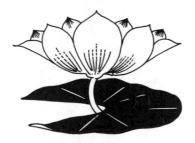

The lotus is another symbol for women's genitals, which is drawn around the edge of yantras, visualization aids. The symbol for the yoni is a triangle, encircled by 16 lotus petals. Lotus petals are often visualized in the location of chakra energy centres (see page 37–9) – they represent the harmonious unfolding of enlightenment. The place associated with enlightenment at the crown of the body map of energy is depicted as a thousand-petal lotus, representing the full flowering of the individual into enlightenment.

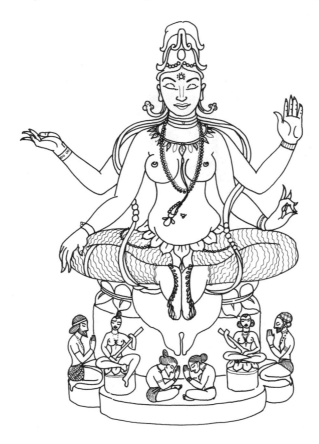

For yoni worship the vulva of a woman, or a sculpted representation of a yoni is worshipped.

Lingam is the sanskrit term for phallus, and it's always depicted erect. The erect lingam represents the focussed awareness of consciousness. According to writer Nik Douglas, it also stands for the universe in a state of excitement – in response to the tantalizing play of dynamic Shakti energy. The phallus has long been worshipped as a fertility symbol. In its erect state it is a celebration of male potency and virility, and a symbol of creativity and courage. The erect phallus stands for the masculine consciousness of Shiva and the retention of semen in Tantric ritual sex.

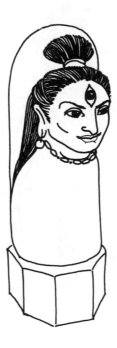

Tantrics say that inside every lingam is a yoni, and inside every yoni is a lingam – the two are inseparable. Both genitals are complementary and connected. Just as Shakti and Shiva are always entwined, so too are the yoni and lingam, represented all over India by carved yoni-lingam sculptures, representing the lingam arising out of a yoni.

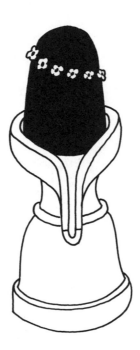

Part 2:
Day-to-Day Tantra

'Woman is the creator of the universe,
the universe is her form; woman is the foundation of the world,
she is the true form of the body.
Whatever form she takes, whether of a man or of a woman,
is the superior form.'

From the Shakti Sangama Tantra

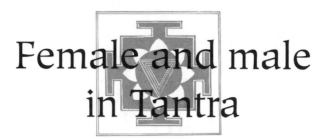

Female and male in Tantra

Dorothy, 39: Getting involved with Tantra has been life-changing for me. I always thought I was very open and liberal, but having been educated at a private Catholic school where there was lots of shame about our bodies and stigma about touching them, I hadn't realized I had so many issues that have been covered up for years. In a workshop for women, we undressed and looked at each others' bodies, which was absolutely amazing. I realized that all women are exactly the same – as well as being so different.

I feel much more in touch with my own body and my own sexuality. I'm not frightened of my sexuality now. I realize it's an incredibly powerful, beautiful thing I've been given. All those powerful experiences I had as a teenager – they were all my own. I'm really happy with my body and my sexuality now. I'm happy with understanding the energy that runs through my body, and I feel more in tune with the universe.

Tantra honours the feminine in both men and women, and acknowledges the creative power represented by women. Women's sexuality is extremely powerful – cultures like those of the Middle East have always known this, and hence attempt to constrain or regulate women. As a result of sexual repression over thousands of years, many women have lost touch with our sexual confidence. For many of us, sexuality is an area fraught with taboos, and many of us get through our early years of ambivalent sexual experiences by splitting this area off from the rest of our lives.

For men, first intercourse is connected with entering manhood, and is wrapped up with complex feelings about power. Men learn about sex through masturbation, and from books and films – especially porn films – all of which represent men as doing things to women, setting up a correlation between masculine sexuality and activity, feminine sexuality and passivity.

In this culture, men generally initiate women into lovemaking. Most women's early experiences are not about sharing our bodies in a state of love – but are about being penetrated, and discovering how to please our partners. We don't learn about love-making from other women, but from our early lovers, from books and films. Then we tend to repeat this learned behaviour, rather than wondrously exploring our bodies anew each time we make love, or with each new lover. Sex has become limited and genitally based, so that many of us continue to make love in the unsatisfying ways that our first lovers taught us. Men feel stuck with the connection between phallic proficiency and power – or grapple with feelings of inadequacy.

Mark, 41: It's always been excruciating for me having a small penis. When I was in my thirties a new lover told me she couldn't bear to carry on because my penis was too small for her. I felt utterly diminished and humiliated. All the awful feelings I'd struggled with in my teens came back to haunt me, and it took me a while to risk taking my clothes off with a lover.

When my partner created a ritual honouring my lingam, it took me ages to relax and let go of my fear of it all going wrong. She was very playful and garlanded my penis with a daisy chain, singing little poems she made up on the spot, which helped relax me. I started to enjoy it, and even found my fears funny. The laughter was healing, and she helped me to appreciate the different moods of my lingam. It doesn't just have to give sexual pleasure, because we can create pleasure between us in so many ways.

Both women and men tend to bring just our genitals into bed, leaving outside our capacity for whole-body sensuality, as well as our intense emotions and our spirituality.

We can compensate for sexual boredom and frustration in several ways – most often by giving up on love-making altogether, or sometimes by getting into a continuous search for greater and greater stimulus, in whatever form we can find it. Whatever our sexual histories, there is often much healing that needs to happen before we can fully explore a Tantric perspective. Much of the new Tantra training currently available in the West addresses this area of sexual healing, as a preparation for Tantra (see page 182–91 – yoni healing and lingam healing).

Arleen, 49: One of the themes of the women's workshop was unravelling the messages our mothers gave us. I realized that my mother had told me by word and deed that being a woman was all about looking after men — well, not just men in general, but a very special man. For her, it was my father, and I'd translated that to mean that a woman's role in life was to look after a special man. She hardly wore any make-up and wore sensible clothes, she never told me or showed me that it was fun being a woman. When I had my first period, she was insistent that I shouldn't tell anyone else about it, that it was a secret.

Hilary gave us the opportunity to re-invent the past.

Taking the idea that it was never too late to have a happy childhood, I re-invented my first period, with my make-believe mother and aunt making a fuss over me, painting my nails and mouth red, saying that this would show the whole world that I was now a woman. OK, this was only make-believe, like a positive form of psychodrama — but it has had a lasting effect on me. A few days after the workshop I went on a shopping spree, treating myself to new makeup for the first time in years. As I speak, my nails are shimmering with purple nail varnish with gold glitter and I can taste the luscious red lipstick I bought, just for me, just for the fun of it.

Tantra is unique in celebrating female sexuality, and making it central to the most advanced spiritual practices. Women have always been pivotal in the history of Tantra – as teachers, initiators and fellow searchers with men. Women often initiated men into Tantric knowledge and the art of transforming sexual pleasure into spiritual ecstasy. Nineteenth century travellers to Tibet described Tantric monks as hermits, living in caves except for visits from their teacher. They meditated on sexual union with her, as a manifestation of the goddess, when she was absent.

While all humans are divine, in Tantric cosmology the feminine principle of creation is considered primary. In love-making she is the active party, who invites her lover to pleasure her, and to enter her, when the time is right for her. The ability to perceive divinity is a mark of progress for both men and women on the Tantric path. The willingness of male practitioners to honour women as the means to their own enlightenment is thought to be particularly crucial to their spiritual progress. According to academic Miranda Shaw, men were expected to worship and serve their Tantric companions.

In any culture that is biased towards men, this apparent sub-servience serves to balance the inner male and female energies. Stepping into this role was, and is, an important way for men to open up to the feminine qualities of their 'inner woman'.

Leone, 29: When I met my partner, I was more in touch with my masculine side, and he was more in touch with his feminine side. He's better at domestic things like cooking and home-making, and he's more receptive and loving than I am. He's better at just being, rather than doing. He also enjoyed make-up and clothes – he cross-dressed – and that persona was playful, flirty and sluttish.

I was the achiever, the doer – and I used to initiate love-making all the time. My sexual energy was voracious. I was always taking my pleasure on top of him, rubbing myself on his stiff penis. Eventually I got fed up and tried to restrain myself. I realize I was trying to control sex. I got in touch with the wounded feminine side of myself, the side that hadn't been able to say no before, that always had to be sexy and didn't look after myself in sex. I realized I didn't always have to have something ramming its way inside me.

I realized we could talk about what we wanted, and I began to allow him on top of me, and to relax more. One time we'd been touching each other gently, and then he entered me very, very slowly. I felt like he was huge – his lingam coming in at this miniscule pace. It felt like his loving energy was coming into me, I felt loved and very safe. I cried with that experience; allowing myself to just trust and let go.

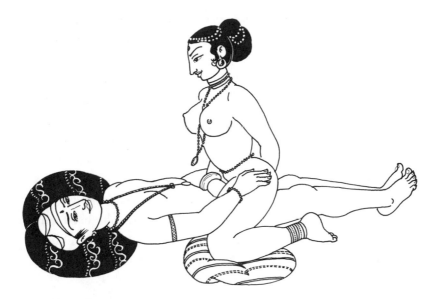

Tantra is geared towards heterosexual relationships, although not exclusively so. Its main ritual use is the female-male dyad. Through uniting the two poles of male and female, our dualistic experience of the world is transformed into one of unity. Tantra uses the idea of bringing lunar and solar energies, negative and positive charges together to harmonize the body both internally and externally. This is why ritual sex is considered so important as a pathway to the Tantric goal of non-duality.

> **Darren, 48:** Being a 100% gay man with lots of sexual experience, it's strange that I've only ever had Tantric experiences when working with a woman. While Tantric techniques have helped me to achieve more intimacy, getting away from what I call 'dick sex' with men, which is just genital, I have only felt that blissful energy working with a woman.
>
> I decided to confront the fear of women that I think all gay men have – the devouring, destructive Kali energy that

threatens to annihilate my sex. I worked with someone who was able to let me go as slowly as I wanted, so I could deal with my fear.

We were sitting cross-legged in front of each other, touching and exploring each other's bodies, and when I felt ready, we Included our genitals in these long, slow sweeps. After a while we did some arousing breathing together – breathing in together with a short, sharp breath, and then slowly relaxing the lungs to let the breath out. This breathing created a much deeper connection between us, and we were able to lie down and stroke each other. She used her hair, her fingertips, her breath, her mouth. I could feel her confident, bold energy, and I was surprised to find myself feeling aroused instead of scared.

Usually if a man is stimulating me the arousal begins in my balls, whereas with her my whole body was feeling aroused, and my genital excitement was almost incidental. I just stopped thinking about what was going on and planning what I was going to do, and surrendered to the experience. I felt a feeling of just being, very relaxed, and then my whole body began to buzz.

Afterwards I felt great for days; happy, bouncy and more balanced, just great on every level.

Rob, 37: I imagined my inner woman. I imagined myself as a woman being made love to by myself, and imagined my yoni. I felt like I had a yoni, it was a real feeling, and strangely appropriate. I felt made whole by this feeling I had a woman inside of me. It was soft, being a woman and powerful. It was a deep experience. She felt like my lover Nina, like a perfect lover, and she was also me, all rolled into one.

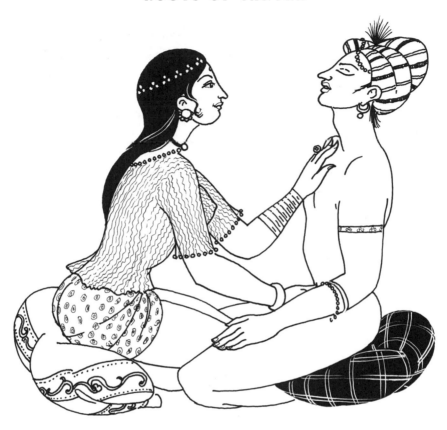

As well as unifying active and passive, masculine and feminine poles externally, it is important to balance and unify them internally. If you're working solo using Tantric exercises, you can visualize an inner lover to create an energetic circle internally.

While we know there is a range of different qualities within us, identifying ourselves exclusively with one gender limits us. We over-emphasize the qualities we associate with our own gender, and undervalue the opposite qualities. These qualities become internalized, associated with what psychoanalyst Jung would call our inner man (if we are a woman) or our inner woman (if we are a man).

The idea of our inner man and inner woman has been used by Tantra to access cut off aspects of ourselves. Working with a partner of the other sex, or using polarized energies, means we can unite with the other half of ourselves by coming together.

Indian sculptures sometimes depict this as Ardhanarisvara, the hermaphrodite god, who is half man and half woman.

In Tantra, the Moon is associated with the left side of the body, feminine energy, cooling quality, the colour white, the element of water and the intuitive processes. Lunar energy is stored at the third-eye chakra, and is depicted in a crescent-shaped moon. The Sun is associated with the right side of the body, masculine energy, the element of fire, the colour red, and intellect. Solar energy is stored in the solar plexus chakra. The union of the two can be accomplished meditatively through visualization.

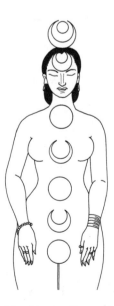

Lunar energy is associated with white, cooling, water Shakti and intuition. Solar energy is associated with the colour red, fire, heat, Shiva and consciousness.

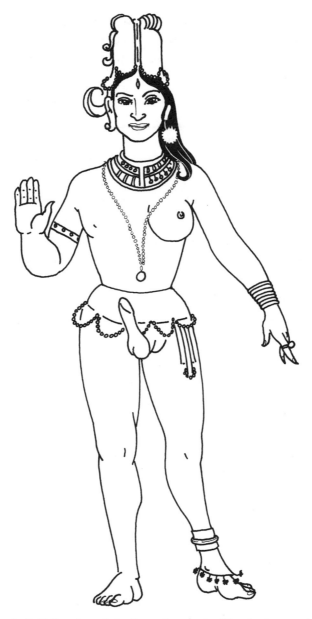

The half male half female god Ardhanarisvara signifies the integration and completion of masculine and feminine.

Bill, 47: I can't imagine going back to the old way of making love. In spite of the loving feelings and good times it was so limited and boring, doing the same things over and over again.

It wasn't nourishing – now I see it was more like a quick wank even with my partner.

The way I make love now feels like a relief. I feel I don't have to perform, and I'm not overly focused on satisfying my partner. I felt an obligation to give my partner an orgasm – she didn't often have one, and I felt it was my fault that I wasn't skilled enough as a lover. Or I felt I didn't get it right in interpreting what she wanted me to do. Now, I realise we weren't communicating properly ver-bally, she didn't let me know how she wanted to be plea-sured or share what was going on for her.

Perhaps she wasn't enough in touch with her own body to be able to tell me. Sometimes we just weren't connected. Now I can spot when my partner goes into her head – it just doesn't work when you're not connected. I need to be in eye contact with my partner, and if I feel her going off into thoughts and fantasies I just ask her to speak out loud all the thoughts that are going through her head – that's usually enough to help us reconnect.

Communication is important in a Tantric relationship. And because I don't have to second guess what she wants I can pay attention to myself.

I can still get excited and play with that excitement, but whereas my excitement used to drop away the minute we stopped sex, now I can stop and I'm still experiencing the excitement without having to keep moving inside her. It's not just my lingam, I'm aware of my whole body and I'm connected with her.

I've learnt through Tantra that I experience more plea-sure by not trying to do anything, and by not trying to achieve orgasm, than I did before. I can follow what my body wants to do in the way of spontaneous movements – it's letting go and surrendering to the actual experience.

And it's surrendering to not being dominant, and not feel-ing I have to do something or make something happen.

That allows my partner to set the pace. If it was up to me I'd speed up, and that's too fast for her.

It's been a process of learning to slow down and stay with the slowness to fit in with her pace.

In surrendering to her pace it has become much more pleasurable for me. I don't even want to rev it up.

It's like a dance of energies. In being able to let go, and keep letting go the energy can change and as she becomes more and more receptive I can be moved to doingness again. I feel I'm leading but it arises naturally out of what's happening between us rather than me doing it automati-cally. It becomes a conscious choice whether I either let go or become active. And when she's fully receptive to my active mode I feel much more pleasure. When she gets more pleasure, I get more pleasure.

Often I don't have a physical orgasm, I used to feel tired and sleepy after ejaculation most nights. Now I come only every couple of weeks – and when I do ejaculate it doesn't diminish my energy.

Tina, 36: I'm much more present during sex now. Before doing Tantra I wasn't really there, I wasn't experiencing sex at the time it was happening. I'd enjoy fantasizing about it when my partner was long gone, but the actual experience wasn't that engaging.

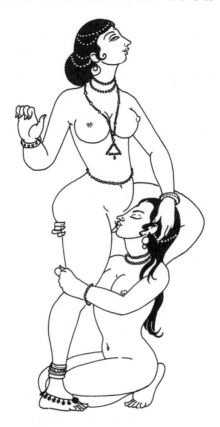

Now I don't feel it's about what I'm doing to my partner or she's doing to me, it's about what's happening to both of us. I'm trying to switch my head off.

I didn't think I was orgasmic, now I find I can let go on another level. I used to ejaculate only at the end of making love, now it happens all the time. At first I thought I was weird, ejaculating.

Lesbian sex is more Tantric anyway, because it's more experimental, without an obvious end. There's no text-book way that you're supposed to make love. The focus on penetration in Tantra doesn't bother us – it's all about how you interpret it. It's really a penetration of energy, and about playing with different kinds of energy. Taking on different roles brings out a different kind of energy in you.

Play is a good way of breaking through your relationship issues – keeping everything lighter. We love to play, erotic play, body painting, dressing up, dancing. It's all about having more fun, and more spontaneous times.

People who love sex love it because it feels good, and it makes them feel good about themselves. Sexuality is integral to the quality of our lives, enhancing, enriching and adding meaning to existence. It's about openness, connectedness and growth, not about one person doing something to another. It's a voyage of mutual discovery and pleasure.

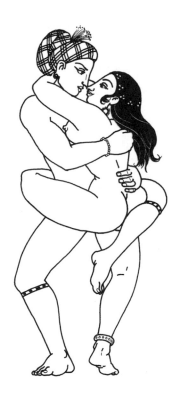

One of the most difficult things for us to learn is to simply say yes to pleasure. Tantra gives you permission to explore your hedonistic side, and to indulge your senses, in the pursuit of everyday ecstasy. Not through mind-altering substances, (although Tantric practitioners have used alcohol and cannabis in their rituals), but through learning to use pleasure as a way of unlocking your own mind. Pleasure is a way of freeing yourself from a joyless existence, and waking up to the sheer joy and divine grace of being alive.

The joy of being alive means living each moment to the full – as if it were your last. Not deferring pleasure and delight until some later date, but trying to squeeze the maximum pleasure from doing whatever it is you're doing – even if it does seem mundane. The idea is not to do anything because of some reward it will bring later, but because you're enjoying it for its own sake. This is part of the Tantric concept of goallessness, particularly in sex. It fosters an attitude of pleasure in the moment, of fully experiencing the present moment rather than trying to make something happen, or worrying about what comes next. This is why it's particularly important to try and let go of the goal of orgasm.

Tantrics don't consider orgasm the goal of sex. The function of sex is as a gateway to experiencing unity, which encompasses unity with the divine. While there are many other tools for enlightenment, sexual practices are considered the most powerful tool in Tantra. While you can still practise Tantra and be celibate, sexual practice acts as a spur to spiritual development, speeding enlightenment.

THE BODY AS A TEMPLE

Marion, 50: For me, it was a big revelation that you didn't have to be fat and have straight hair to hate your body, even model-slim women with curly hair have problems. I'd spent a lifetime believing that happiness came with curly hair – and here were goddesses incarnate complaining about having to iron their hair so that it would look straighter! Women with beautiful long legs and slender figures listing all the things they hated about their bodies – I couldn't believe my ears!

When it was my turn it was easy enough to strip off and talk about all the things I disliked about my body – my fat tummy and huge thighs – but it was much harder to talk about the things I liked. Well, yes, I do quite like my ears, and my strong hands, oh yes and I've been told I've got such lovely blue eyes that they must be alright. But it was even more difficult to stand up naked in front of two beautiful women who gave me honest feedback about my body – my beautiful breasts, my classical contours, my firm muscle tone, my perfect proportions. Hilary encouraged me to carry on breathing, and to really listen to what the other women were saying.

Many women are literally outside themselves, not daring to inhabit their bodies. We don't feel comfortable in our bodies because of the cultural messages we receive throughout our lifetime which prevent us from revelling in them, whatever shape or size we are, and from enjoying the experiences our bodies bring us.

It is rare to see a young woman who revels in her body, with the pure celebratory joy of just being alive. Young women in our

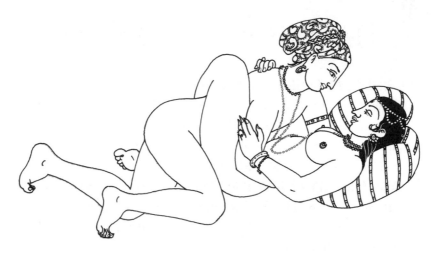

culture don't learn how to be in their own power sexually, and it's a long journey before they feel they can be themselves, rather than what media images, peer pressure and men want them to be. Many of us do not come into a sense of our own sexual power until our mid-thirties, when we already have a lot of negative experiences that need to be released or healed in some way. Many women say they become mothers before becoming women.

Men also have a difficult relationship with their sexual power, often feigning a virility that masks a lack of confidence underneath. Our culture expects men to assume a dominant sexuality, pursuing potential mates and initiating sex, yet it castigates men for doing just that. Many men carry a lot of fear and insecurity over their sexual prowess and find it just as hard to inhabit their bodies as women do. A Tantric attitude is to see the beauty of each aspect of life in a non-judgmental way and meet everything in an attitude of respect. Anything that rejects the body rejects the innate beauty of the person, and in that sense is anti-Tantric.

Rob, 37: A lot of shame has been healed doing Tantra. I've always had shame about my body. I hated my body. The way it looks. I've always felt pudgy, and there were a couple of experiences at boarding school where I was humiliated when I was naked. One was in the changing rooms at school and another time was when my brother and his friend ridiculed me. I'm very embarrassed about my genitals, and I've always hated changing rooms and toilets. I'd never confronted it and felt so released after doing a strip in front of the group. My body has freed up – I've even been able to dance naked.

For those of us who have problems relating sexually in this culture of repression and denial, sexual healing is needed to free sexual energy from its distortions, and associations with power and violence. This traditionally masculine need for power over another person is replaced by a more mutual way of framing a relationship, based on care and respect.

Too many of us have been going through the motions sexually. Many of us experience deep dissatisfaction around our sex lives. We are looking for real intimacy and tenderness, and deep connection.

Gary, 39: When my lingam is being massaged, I can completely let go, and allowing someone else to play with it can create a real sense of abandonment. Otherwise I can feel my penis is a weapon. I feel a lot of aggression and power and I have to restrain that. I battle with wanting to take complete control – wanting to pin them down and use the lingam to penetrate. That's with either a man or a woman, but for a man to subjugate himself to me is much more exciting. It's as if my brain has gone to my lingam, and it feels like a natural thing to do with this hard thing.

According to Tantra practitioner Charlotte Koelliker, reclaiming the sensitivity of the body is important for healing. In healing there is a real honouring of both the woman and the man, and a development of a more feminine approach to sexuality, redressing the male dominated approach that has reigned up till now. Tantric techniques are ideal, with their emphasis on pleasure, on taking time, on really feeling and experiencing what is happening, and on awakening the whole body to pleasure.

During advanced Tantric rituals, deities are invited into the sacred space set up by the couples, through the use of mudras (gestures), mantras (invocations) and visualizations. The body is transformed by these rituals into a temple space for the divine. Just as the temples in India are seen as specially charged with power – as sites where parts of Shakti's body; the yoni, nipples, and tongue, landed after her disembodiment according to one myth – so the body can be charged up by visualizing deities in various locations.

Nyasa (literally placing), is the ritual used for transforming the physical body into a mirror of the divine by gesturing the location of deity attributes in the body of your partner. While touching energetically charged areas of the body – including your partner's eyes, nostrils, mouth, arms and thighs – deities, yantras or lotuses are visualized.

THE WAY OF PLEASURE

Leone, 29: On holiday, David was licking my pearl very gently, with a very soft touch, while I was lying very relaxed. I felt very trusting, I felt as if I didn't have to communicate what was happening to me, I could just go inside. All sorts of images were coming into my mind. It was like a kaleidoscope of different colours. This light touch on my

pearl felt very healing, and it enabled me to go into my consciousness in a pleasurable way; loving and expansive.

After love-making we were eating together in the same
room. There was still a tangible sense of energy in the
room. We were doing everything very slowly. We were
feeding each other very slowly. We both became watery
eyed, because every movement we made seemed so beautiful to us. It was almost conscious, as if we could see ripples
made by each movement. With our eye contact we felt
immediately transported into another place. A place of
extreme sensitivity. A place of great well-being, where we
could just rest. It was an experience of love.

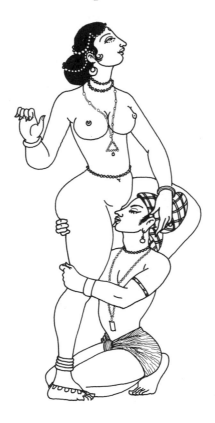

In a Tantric relationship it is important to acknowledge your entitlement to pleasure. Pleasure is your birthright, and its greatest enemy is all-too-common feelings of shame and guilt around the body. Developing sensual enjoyment is central to the Tantric approach to life. Rather than try to subjugate desire through repression, Tantra teaches us to cultivate the art of living in this world as if it were sacred. Everyday awareness cannot evolve unless we experience everyday life in its full power.

The Tantric view is that it is not the world that is limited, it is our way of looking at it. Enlightened beings experience the world as a place of bliss, while us unenlightened mortals experience the world as suffering. This is why Tantra places such a premium on identifying and incorporating deity into our self, believing that what we focus our attention on determines what we experience.

Therefore Tantra is not concerned with identifying with emotions, which oscillate between positive and negative. Far too many of us get stuck in negative patterns. Feelings, (which are linked to sensations) rather than emotions (which are linked to thoughts), are the main means of developing Tantric awareness. Feelings are about being connected with the world, or with another. They are about being truly present, in each moment, to whatever experience has to offer. Feeling (or sensation) is cultivated rather than thinking, because thoughts tend to dilute or destroy the directness and intensity of experience. Tantrics focus and develop feeling through paying attention to the sensations discovered by their five senses.

In Indian thought the idea of play implies a conscious spiritual self for whom play is a delightful way of sporting with reality. Since reality is the dance of creation, we should learn to dance with it. Natural play is that which stimulates and nourishes the five senses. The senses are delighted and stimulated through offerings, flowers, lights, incense and chimes, and delicate essences such as rosewater.

EMOTIONS

Ann, 49: We spent the morning talking about our hopes and fears for the weekend. I explained that I was alone and for the first time in my life I was no-one's daughter, no-one's lover. My partner had just left me for a much younger woman. Apparently you're as young as the lover you're with. My fear was that I'd spend the whole weekend crying – my hope was to experience ecstasy. I was comforted by John telling me that all my emotions were part of the same process of becoming whole. He said: 'In Tantra it's OK to cry, it's OK to have any emotion, Tantra is about flowing from one emotion to another.'

Later in the weekend I understood what he meant when we did the 'moving centre' exercise. We walked around the room, then John told us to explore various emotions for a minute or two, and then switch to neutral again, simply walking. It was delightful to have permission to be really angry with someone, and then move on, calm down, spend a moment or two with myself and then to be tender, gently stroking someone's face.

The path of relationship in Tantra is not the path of emotions. The Tantric path is not a psychotherapy path that elevates emotions into our guiding *raison d'être*. Nor does it advocate control of emotions. Instead, whichever emotions come and go can be watched without much passion, excitement or even interest. This requires a degree of detachment from emotions, their causes and the possible outcomes that we hope to effect through them.

Everything is in a state of flux, including our emotional states. Emotions come and go, changing and disappearing almost as soon as they arise. Using meditation and other Tantric techniques, you can learn to hold your own internal centre as these states come and go, not getting sucked into your emotions, or identifying yourself with your current emotional state.

All emotion is simply energy – it is our limited, dualistic way of thinking that casts emotions as negative or positive. If we are stuck in our emotions, and the scenarios we create in our minds, we can't be free to truly experience our energy body. We are stuck in the limitations of our mind.

The fundamental principle of Tantra is that spiritual progress cannot be made through repressing shadow aspects and negative emotions, but by actively transforming them. Tantra is not concerned with stilling emotions, but with not being attached to emotions – or to outcomes.

Dealing with emotions

Ariane, 38: I was always frightened of Des. He seemed to exude aggression and apparently his pent-up frustration had occasionally erupted in violence in his relationships.

I avoided working with him on my training course, in spite of the Tantric ethos of trying to step beyond personality issues and connect with the essentially divine being in front of you.

One day I found myself sitting cross-legged in front of Des, to do a fire meditation. As we started deep breathing and visualizing flames in our base chakras, I felt put off by the intensity of his laboured breathing. Even his breathing seemed aggressive to me.

'And as Shiva he should be following my pattern of breathing!' I thought. I started to withdraw, feeling intimidated by his overbearing presence.

But then the Tantric adage clicked in my head. 'It's all just energy.' While he might sometimes express it as anger or violence, Des was sitting on a powder-keg of energy. And I'm a powerful person too. The way to meet him on an energy level was not to follow my usual inclination to retreat and make myself smaller, but to manifest my own power.

I breathed deeply into my pelvis, allowing the energy in my base chakra to expand, and ignite, using the image of flames to help me. Eyes closed, I went inside to get in touch with my own power.

Suddenly the flame caught and I could feel the heat building up around my sitting bones. I opened my eyes and looked directly into Des's eyes as we both breathed together, our energies alive and suddenly dancing together, all fear and holding back gone.

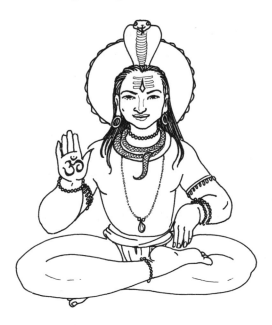

As well as learning to celebrate sexuality, Tantra encourages you to take things lightly in your relationship, and not get sucked into difficult negative emotional patterns. For instance, not responding to rows and conflicts with destructive 'this is the end of the relationship' scenarios. Finding a Tantric way of dealing with emotional difficulties involves making a commitment to shifting out of negative emotional states, rather than allowing them to fester and damage the quality of communication in your partnership.

The path to enlightenment involves transforming the emotions of desire, fear and anger in particular. According to traditional Tantrics, those unable to cut the knots of shame, hate and fear are not worthy of initiation into this path. In order to experience love we need to drop fear. In order to connect, we need to drop anger and blaming. In order to surrender, we need to let go of our desires. Tantra offers practical tools to work at transmuting fear and attachment into love and universal power.

> *Bill, 47*: I had to revise my own internal concepts of masculinity – letting go of how I thought I should behave and embracing more pleasure. I don't really have a model of the masculine now – it becomes irrelevant when you're working with energies.
>
> Originally I was afraid of expressing my anger, and afraid of what I thought being a man was all about. Talking with other men was really helpful, as well as thinking about the oedipal triangle I had with my parents.
>
> In the couples session on the training course we enacted a typical argument with our partner, where we looked at our patterns of just blaming each other – that's helped me to stop doing it.

I've allowed my partner to teach me the language of emotions because she was much more used to expressing herself because of the psychotherapy she'd done in the past.

I found the Tantric model of following the women's pace and rhythm helpful, and ultimately more relaxing and satisfying.

Teacher Hilary Spenceley says that people who embark on Tantra as a path of self-development need to have done some psychological work on themselves, before being able to fully grasp the spiritual learning implicit in Tantra.

For instance, you need to be aware of your tendency to project your own emotions and issues onto others, and to have developed ways of staying with whatever is going on – even when things get tough. Whether you're crying, angry, fearful or blaming, all these emotions are your own. In order to get through them she suggests that you stay with them, rather than running away from them. It's a challenge to take responsibility for your own emotions and not to feel either victimized or blaming about anything that comes up. Otherwise, you will end up constantly fighting with and blaming your partner as you attempt Tantric practices together. Tantric techniques can enable you to get to a point where you can treat these emotions as pure energy, rather than anything real.

Instead, you can learn to concentrate on feelings and sensation. Emotions are our ego response to the things that happen to us, while feelings are our sensory experience of the things that are happening to us. Feelings are very much to do with the present, while emotions tend to have roots in the past. Instead of sapping your energy because you're reliving and recreating old emotional traumas, feelings are fresh and energizing. If you feel you're getting into an emotional tangle, you can do a 'reality check' – concentrate on what's really going on right now with the person in front of you, rather than what you think is going on. Relaxing back into the sense of contact and connection between you can help more love to come in, and keep you out of defensive or attacking angry mode with your partner.

Sylvie, 50: I've let go of the idea that being sexual was condemning me to the fire of hell ... I am striving to let go of my ideas about romantic love, and any notion that I am entitled to anything from my lover just because we are lovers.

I'm also letting go of the idea that intimacy is easy. In two marriages lasting over 25 years, we just moved in together and thought we could sail into the sunset.

I'm trying to let go of all my ideas about what a relationship should or shouldn't be.

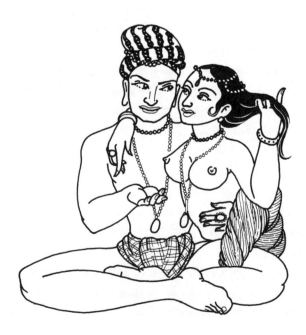

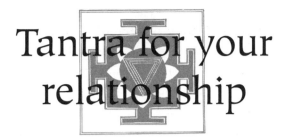

Tantra for your relationship

Dorothy, 39: In spite of a good relationship, after 18 years our sex life is often boring. It's part of the culture that men have to be very geared into performance, and are so much into penetration. It's all about how long penetration lasts, and there isn't that sense of touch and stillness. I want to do Tantra with my partner to take our sexual relationship onto a whole other level.

I think we have a great relationship, kids, houses and a business. But we did a weekend for couples recently, during which I cried inconsolably for hours. I don't know why, I was just releasing emotion because of a huge sense of relief at being given permission just to be there. My partner spontaneously told everyone present how he felt witnessing his wife's emotional outpouring; 'I've realized Dorothy and I had become very disconnected over the years, and how connected we've just become. I can't wait for more.

Many couples in long-term relationships face the question of how to rekindle the erotic spark, while others complain of unfulfilled longings for tenderness and love in the performance culture of today's sexuality. The pressure to perform means that our sexuality remains limited, genitally focused. The way we view sex, and its place in our relationships, needs changing. By construing touch as a sexual invitation we miss out on affectionate touch and our senses are starved. By focusing on the mechanics of sexual techniques and positions our creativity is stifled and the potential for increasing intimacy is lost. Relationships can become negative and constricting – and unsensual!

Contemporary approaches to sexuality are very restricted. Practitioners of Tantra maintain that by transforming the context of sex, we can transform the experience. Tantric exercises focus on vitality, sensuality and relationship rather than sexuality in the limited way we usually understand it. Tantric approaches are not concerned so much with what we do, but with the way we do it. Love-making is not so much about technique, it's about approaching your lover with a heart filled with love – as the Beloved, as the divine.

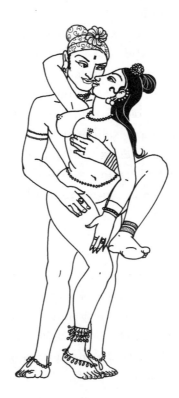

According to Tantra teacher John Hawken, a typically neurotic relationship dynamic is where two beggars, clinging together out of fear and neediness, play power games to persuade or force the other to finally come up with the emotional goods — which they haven't got themselves because they feel empty.

Tantric techniques can support each individual in discovering their own desires; stepping out of a victim mentality by experiencing oneself as the source of one's own pleasure and taking responsibility for one's own fulfilment. Each couple needs to find ways of relating which are more sensual than sexual. The trust between a couple makes it possible to heal old wounds, fears and blocks. Instead of focusing on the failings of our partner and not understanding why they won't give us what we need, we need to approach them with a sense of our own dignity, worth and fullness of experience.

CREATING A
TANTRIC RELATIONSHIP

John Hawken, Tantra teacher: What we call love in our society is often more about neediness — we say 'I love you', meaning 'I need you'. We are brought up to believe that the source of love is outside ourselves. There's also a false understanding of how energy works. Our society sees love according to material rules rather than energetic rules. For instance, we have the feeling there is only a certain amount of love to go round. 'If someone else is getting it that means there is less for us.' 'If I give it away, I have less.' And so we learn to hoard love, but because love is an energy it doesn't work like that at all. We don't gain extra energy by holding onto it. The more we have, the more we keep it flowing. So it's not something that gets used up.

A Tantric paradigm of relationship is that we come together as king and queen, out of an overflowing and full-ness. 'I'm compete in myself, but because of the joy of experiencing myself in the flowing it's great to come and share the experience with you.'

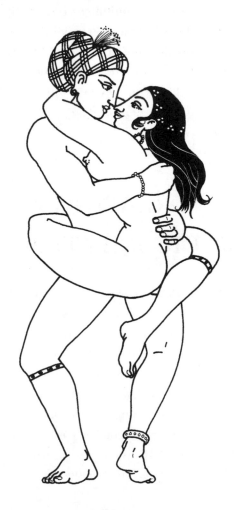

In a typical relationship we try to relate to each other as adults, but often get caught up in the childish part of ourselves, or the parenting part, depending on the dynamic of the relationship. We tend to get enmeshed in our own and others' histories, traumas, and dramas – the soap operas of our lives. In a Tantric relationship you are trying to let go of the historical story that forms your personality over your lifetime – the personal 'ego'. Instead you are trying to relate to one another on the level of the divine. You discover your energy body and its potential by letting go again and again of who you think you are and what you identify with, and becoming more than that. Tantra says you are more than the sum of your parts. And your relationship is more than the sum of your two personalities.

A Tantric relationship is one in which you're trying to spend as much time as possible connected together in Shakti-Shiva energy. What's going on in day-to-day life is only important because of the energetic charge that these dramas create in us. These energetic residues need to be cleared, or transformed in order to step into a sacred space with our partner.

The more you can step into a sacred space with your partner, the more a sense of the divine becomes the foreground in the relationship rather than something background that is occasionally dipped into. Because Tantra is a core discipline, with core values, incorporating it into your relationship requires constant attention – it's not just about spicing up your bedroom routine. Purification is an essential part of preparing to meet the other – your divine lover – in the realm of the divine, without the murkiness of emotional baggage and neediness.

Sexual rituals in Tantra are about creating an energetic connection, rather than fulfilling emotional needs. It's about a mingling of the red (shakti) and white (shiva) energies in each person and between a couple – but not a merging. Each colour is distinct and powerful in its own right, but open to the enrichment that comes through the meeting of energies.

One of the things that is so appealing about Tantric philosophy is that there's no right or wrong. Of course, this is precisely where those who are not conscious can get trapped by Tantra's obvious seductiveness, because you need to develop your own sense of alignment with divinity rather than having it mapped out and road-marked for you.

The actual form of your relationship is completely up to you both, but you need a strong connection in order to really go deep. There is no sense in which a non-committed relationship can be fully Tantric. It's a path of authenticity, integrity and wholeness.

According to Charlotte Koelliker, Tantra practitioner, to create a Tantric relationship you need:

- consciousness about working with energy

- to come together out of complete mutual respect and freedom understanding that you're together to give each other pleasure

- to bring sex and consciousness together

- to realize that the divine is in the other, and to want to connect with it

- commitment to being honest and truthful as you can about your own emotional issues

- commitment to working towards greater consciousness.

What is key to a Tantric relationship is that you both fully acknowledge the sacredness of sexuality, and are able to see that

sexuality can be a spiritual discipline which is capable of transforming your life.

If that is present other things will fall into place. If you're
committed to connecting with the essence of your partner, and
trying not to get caught up in emotional problems that get in the
way, you're well on the way to developing a good Tantric relationship. Nurture your feelings of respect for the person, and
work at disentangling the negative feelings you project onto your
partner. (See exercise page 117 clearing the air.)

This means making space to allow the other person to be
themselves, and accepting them as they are. This involves letting
go of fantasies about the perfect relationship and the perfect
lover. It means being committed to the truth, even when the truth
is painful, but also about being careful about our, at times,
masochistic attachment to pain in relationships.

Tantra requires the courage to let go of conventions and
shoulds and shouldn'ts in relationships, and being willing to go
on a journey into the unknown. It means staying with your partner on this journey through times of confusion and uncertainty
because the path hasn't been mapped out. Just as traditional
Tantrics flouted social norms, being on the Tantric path involves
shedding layers of cultural conditioning about what relationships
should be, and especially about how sex should be. Tantra is
about not being stuck in one way of interacting. It's about having
the freedom to enjoy all aspects, all possibilities and all manifestations. Tantra is about dancing all the possibilities in your relationship. It's a positive statement to commit to exploring all aspects of
your sexuality together. Creative use of ritual is one of the Tantric
methods for encouraging and containing this process of exploration.

TANTRA FOR SEXUAL HEALING

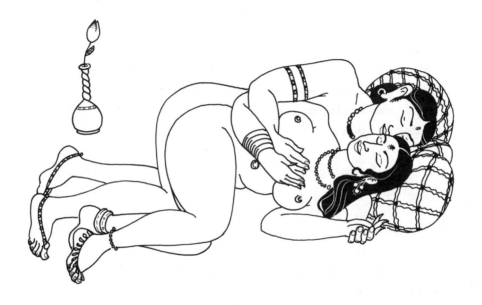

Mavis, 30: Before I used to have problems staying on the ground. That was much worse as a result of abuse I went though in my teens. I used to feel a presence around me all the time – his presence. And I'd just go out of my body to get away.

Since I've been seeing a Tantric therapist with my partner I feel that I do deserve to be honoured. Relating with a sense of sacredness and a heart connection has been very important. It's the sacredness that makes me feel safe. Before I couldn't have sex with my boyfriend. I just felt totally raw and afraid. I'd burst into tears all the time. Now I'm much clearer about my boundaries, I know when I don't feel comfortable with something, rather than telling myself, 'oh well, it doesn't matter' and then suffering for it. I still feel I need to take the lead in the relationship to feel safe, but our relationship has really improved.

When we did the yoni healing exercise, where I was touched in such an intimate but non-sexual way – in a way I never had been touched before, that was really a healing experience.

And one day during a self-love ritual, when I was pleasuring myself, I felt that presence intrude again. Spontaneously I made a ritual to get rid of him, and to get rid of the legacy of the abuse. It was really powerful, and he hasn't been back since. I felt really good about doing that, and I would never have been able to do it without the support of Tantra.

For most of us, the emotional baggage tied up with sex and relationships means that we have to clear a lot of debris, healing sexual wounds and integrating split-off parts of ourselves before we can even start to use sex as a magical means to wholeness and unity. Sex therapy, the medical answer to sexual dissatisfaction, avoids this tricky problem, opting instead for the easier job of promoting more effective sexual techniques. Yet sensible suggestions to schedule time together or to ask for what you want in bed may not always work, because closeness remains elusive if the underlying issues about intimacy are not addressed. Therapists all agree that real intimacy is what we need to explore our full sexual potential. Intimacy is not co-dependency, but a connection between two autonomous beings. It's in a relationship where both individuals are differentiated – different but equal – that we can choose to connect in order to explore these differences creatively.

The most common sexual problem, lack of desire, is particularly responsive to Tantric work. Many couples find that they lose sexual spontaneity in a long-term relationship: spontaneity is replaced by a sense of continuity that can be experienced as habit, and then boredom frequently becomes a problem. Andy, 38, attended a couple of workshops with sex therapists Zak and Misha Halu, before going on to do A Taste of Tantra with SkyDancing. In a relationship for two years, he wanted to avoid the boredom that inevitably set in for him:

> *Andy, 38*: Tantra has meant a gradual change of attitude. I feel less aimed at penetrative sex, full stop. That's no longer an end in itself. I feel there's a whole world of possibilities now.

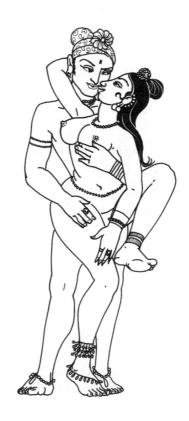

Our natural ability to delight in the senses is dampened by our limited view of sex as an instinctual physical drive.

A common problem for women, for which conventional Masters and Johnson sex therapy approaches often prove woefully inadequate, is inability to orgasm. Sarah, married for 14 years, hadn't been able to reach orgasm for several years. She describes the result of her partner's involvement in the SkyDancing year-long programme:

> *Sarah, 48*: What helped is just relaxing and enjoying the process, instead of trying desperately to reach a climax before my partner comes. He doesn't seem to be bothered about coming, so I no longer feel we're always running out of time. He enjoys my body so much, I can relax and enjoy him enjoying me.

Jenny found that her sexuality closed down after the birth of her first child ten years ago:

> *Jenny, 42:* I had a tear deep in my vagina and anus, which needed loads of stitches, and my whole perineum felt damaged – for years after. I started shutting down sexually, and began feeling really negative about my whole body. Previously sex had been one of the key ways of expressing myself, and without it I felt really stuck.
>
> My partner wasn't really interested, but I went anyway on some Tantric workshops. They took the focus off genital sex and broadened sexuality into sensuality and play. Now, I feel sex is more a whole-body experience, and my body feels much more relaxed. My perineum has finally healed and all the tension I was holding there because of the trauma has melted. Now I can even have orgasms without

any genital stimulation – just by having my nipples, or the rest of my body touched.

There is a lot of shame in our culture, and one of the most common therapeutic results of Tantric workshops is healing sexual shame and guilt.

Derek, 48, a boarding and public school survivor, has done John Hawken's year-long couples training twice, with his partner of 20 years:

Derek: In my twenties I had lots of short relationships. As a man growing up in a public school environment 'having a fuck' was a feather in your cap, something to notch up and then brag about. Sex was very irregular, and quick – something I thought I needed to do to relieve tension. In fact, my whole body felt tense, rigid, dry and unnourished. A lot of the time I didn't feel much. I didn't enjoy my body, and I certainly didn't luxuriate in sex. So for me the training has been a very healing journey, and Tantra feels like the most natural thing in the world.

I've always had a problem with intimacy, and the greatest change has been the improved intimacy in our marriage. I can enjoy my body, and enjoy self-pleasuring, which was always something shameful that I did in private. Someone who masturbates is considered totally ineffectual in life – a real wanker, but through the course a lot of taboos and shame have cleared, leaving me much freer.

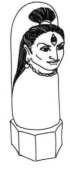

I've worked on oil rigs, building sites and driven trucks and the way we used to treat women out on the streets – whistling and shouting abuse – was so common. That's really turned around now. One of the exercises, where we honour the yoni (female genitals), – which was very hard for me first time round, has become a sacred experience. The whole approach of honouring the feminine has meant reversing the deeply entrenched pattern of seeing women as objects.

In this sense, SkyDancing Tantra is pioneering a new brand of sex therapy – one that focuses on the quality of sex and the relationship between partners – not just physical or psychological, but spiritual as well. For teacher John Hawken, Tantric sex involves coming together, not just 'coming'.

TANTRA IN THE WEST

John Hawken, Tantra teacher: My partner and I started to look for a couples workshop to take part in – we were afraid of joining a mixed open group. Afraid of losing each other, meeting someone better, which you don't have on couples training because everyone has their own partner. It felt like the difference between shark-free and shark-infested waters, but that was the fantasy rather than the reality of the Tantra group. There were lots of rumours about what happened at Tantra groups, and quite a lot of them true. They were much wilder in those days – less Tantric. If you start liberating sexual energy, people usually experience impulses of going over the top – what you'd do if you'd drunk a bottle of champagne, you wouldn't do if you were sober. But Tantra is about liberating the energy and holding the discipline simultaneously. It's like having one foot on the accelerator and one foot on the brake – surrendering in order to experience energetic liberation and abandon but keeping the discipline of honouring oneself and the other, so the energy doesn't become dissipated.

Sophie, 41: I'd just been on a four-day women's retreat, camping on Dartmoor, where we swam together naked, and spent time looking at and appreciating each others' bodies and genitals. It was the first time I'd let in this sense of admiration, and after that I noticed people's perceptions of me had changed. People usually see me as calm, serene and wise, and for the first time a couple of men seemed to find me sexy, and someone fell in love with me. I'd learnt that time spent with your own sex can bring you into contact with your own sexuality.

Feeling this new sense of myself helped me take risks on the Tantra course. During an exercise where we were asked to enter a temple devised by a small group of men, I felt able to leave my fear outside the temple door. I suddenly felt I wanted to take my clothes off, and for the men to take theirs off, and massage me. I noticed that three of the four men had erections, and I was just about to panic when I realized, "No, I'm not going to get raped.": I didn't feel threatened by the men's erections, as I would usually have done. Instead I felt this was great, their erections were due to the effect I was having on them.

This is what I find in Tantra: it shifts you out of a situation you would normally find threatening, because you are feeling powerless or victimized, and allows you to be proactive rather than passive. An example is when I went to Margo Anand's workshop, in which all the women sat as oracles, blindfolded in a circle, waiting to be selected by a Shiva coming to ask a question of us. My mind started worrying "Oh my God, how am I going to handle this?" Using Tantra techniques I breathed, told myself I would handle it. Then my Shiva told me he'd chosen to come to me because I looked like a priestess. So all the time we have an invitation not to go into our fears, but to go into other ways of being.

Workshops in the West combine ancient Tantric practices of Kundalini yoga and meditation with techniques from modern humanistic psychology to develop the ability to connect and communicate with our partners as separate individuals responsible for our own happiness and pleasure. As SkyDancing teacher John Hawken put it; 'Rather than making your partner the object of and focus for your sensual pleasure, you focus on yourself. Your partner is not the cause of or the object of your desire – you are, and you choose how to share that pleasure.'

Most couples come because they're in a relationship that has lost its fire, although they love the other person and want to stay with them. Some couples come because they are fighting and are looking for harmony in their relationship. A lot of singles come because they can't find a partner, so they look at themselves and their sexuality, with the question 'why aren't I attracting a partner? What is it about me that frightens others away?'

Many older people come because they have started on the journey of looking inside themselves, rather than trying to change external situations. There are a lot of wounded people coming on the training, people with abuse stories, and a lot of people who are conscious of their past sexual repression and are looking for healing. As a result of the sexual revolution many of us have experimented with promiscuity and are looking for a deeper sexual revolution, which brings truth and real happiness. There are also a high proportion of inexperienced men who are looking for an initiation into what sexuality is.

In workshops, Tantra gives you a chance of non-genital erotic contact with your partner, or with other people. You can share liveliness and the many other possible qualities that Tantra opens up. You discover there are many beautiful ways of relating to other people, and the compulsion to be genital loses its importance.

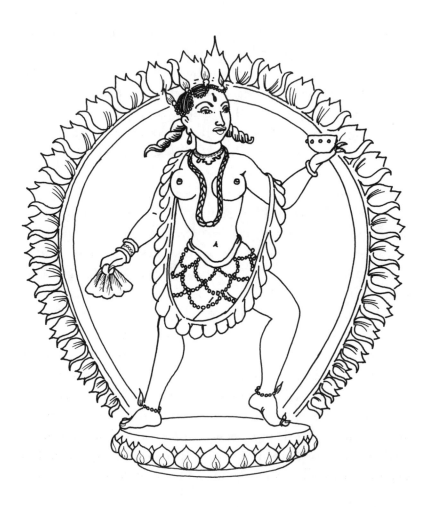

People who have done a Tantric training tend to make love less often than average because as the experience becomes more satisfying it loses its compulsive quality. As the other parts of the body become eroticized, you can experience satisfaction without genital contact.

According to John Hawken, 'In our Tantra groups we try to recreate a sense of innocence, to rediscover the lost innocence of childhood. Innocence is a very important key in opening up our heart so that we no longer do things that are heartless.' Workshops in the West are really preparation for Tantra as a spiritual practice. They work on clearing sexual and emotional blocks and expanding our consciousness of ourselves as energetic beings, while initiating us into a more connected way of relating to each other which opens up our heart. All this is preparation for the spiritual work of aligning ourselves with the divine. For those who want to develop Tantra as a spiritual path, the traditional approach is to find a spiritual teacher who can guide you along the path.

James Low, sex therapist and Tantric Buddhist, has a word of caution about the whole business of Tantra as it's offered in workshops here in Europe:

Tantra is not taught in a traditional way here. It's not a specifically sexual practice in the East, but does use external excitement to focus attention instead of dispersing it. In the East Tantric practices are done only after you've already built up spiritual practices which create a strong ethical framework and after you've undergone a process of purification. This groundwork provides a whole context of clarity and simplicity in which you can start to build up a richness of experience. Through this spiritual discipline you work on your shadow side. In the West people have enormous problems with discipline, and by throwing yourself into erotic practices without looking at your motivations, whether of loneliness, envy, greed or control, you can get caught up in the shadow side of Tantra, merely acting out issues of power and control without challenging them. The Eastern Tantrics always said that the very things that set them free, were the things that snare ordinary people.

Low suggests that there needs to be a balance between *yoga*, 'yoking' oneself to a path of unification, and *Tantra*, which is an aesthetic path of enjoyment and pleasure.

'If you haven't done some form of yoga first, how will you know when there's an imbalance? It needs to be embedded in a sense of purpose.'

Yoga means 'yoke', not the yoke of a work-house bullock, but the voluntary yoke of intention on the path to union with the Divine.

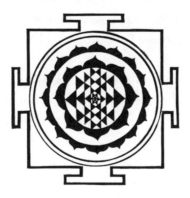

Part 3:
Practical Tantra

'The body is Shakti. The needs of the body are
the needs of Shakti. When man enjoys, it is Shakti
who enjoys through him. His ears, eyes, hands and feet
are Hers. She sees through his eyes, works through
his hands, and hears through his ears. Body, mind,
breath, egoism, intellect, organs and all the other
functions are Her manifestations.'

Swami Sirananda Sarasvati

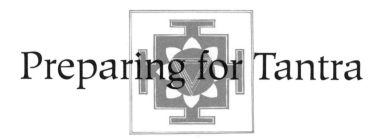

Preparing for Tantra

You can practise most of the following exercises on their own, and then incorporate them at any point in your love-making. When practising solo, if an exercise needs a partner you can invoke a partner by visualizing one. This imaginary lover has a long pedigree in Tantra.

Tantric relationship is about trying to get disciplined: you need to be disciplined to set up sacred space for making love in. It's too easy not to bother, just as it's often easy not to bother with making love at all. It's a good idea to start your exploration of the Tantric path of relationship by building up a practice: set times, say, 'Okay, on Thursday evening at eight we start, each week.' And you start exploring some of these exercises, no matter what mood you're in. Making that commitment in the first place helps you to get into the right mood. As with any practice you need to do it regularly in order for it to have any real effect.

First of all, you need to both agree that this is what you want to do. It's no good one person going along with it for their partner's sake. It is fundamental that both partners should be committed to exploring Tantra together, rather than one person trying to cajole or bully the other person into doing what they want.

For the first few weeks, you can use the time you have committed to spend together to explore preparatory exercises, like meditating at the same time, learning how to connect and honour each other in the tantric way, and setting up your sacred erotic space, in which you will be making love.

Read through the exercises together before you do them and

discuss any changes you might like to make in the exercises I have suggested. Feel free to change things that don't seem appropriate or comfortable for both of you.

Tantra uses techniques of kundalini yoga, breathing, visualization, dance and body work to develop your awareness of your energy body, which in turn leads to cultivating sensuality in its broadest sense. When working with the visualisations suggested, you don't have to see images. Just trust that they are there. Some people sense impressions through feelings, thoughts or through sight, sound, taste or small.

Meditation focuses attention on the chakra energy centres in the body to encourage you to consciously transform your own energy. Tantric exercises and practices are designed to evoke a sense of spirituality, which develops as you incorporate an internal centredness between you both. You need to cultivate silence and stillness as internal quantities in order to allow the experience of ecstasy to emerge.

It's very important to relax before engaging in Tantra, as well as during. Tantric sex is not about releasing the tension you've accumulated throughout the day through getting rid of excess sexual energy, it's about letting go of physical and psychological tension and allowing your sexual energy to flow fully through your body and your energy system.

In this sense it's more about building a positive charge (of energy) rather than getting rid of a negative charge (stress). There are several stages in creating Tantric energy in rituals:

- Relax – let go of stress and tension, and come home to yourself.

- Connect – be in the present moment and connect with your lover in the present moment.

- Build up an energetic charge – through body movement or building up your energy through breathing and visualization techniques.

- Relax into energy charge – sink into the energy you have created.

The same principles apply to sex. For too many of us sex is something we do to unwind – then we turn over and go to sleep. In a Tantric approach sex is a means of creating, exploring, and sustaining intensity of experience. So we need to unwind before we commence making love, in order to connect properly with our partner. You may need to talk about the days events before being able to let go of thinking about them.

That could mean taking a bath – alone or together – to relax, or going out for a walk to clear the debris of the day from your body and mind. It could mean making a nice meal together, and taking the time to consciously appreciate the meal, and eating together.

PREPARING YOURSELF

According to Tantra, both women and men need to purify themselves in order to be able to connect sex and spirit, and to meet on a sacred level. It's important to purify your body through an appropriate lifestyle. Indian Tantrics follow a grain-based vegetarian diet, reserving taboo foods for ritual use. They practise colonic cleansing to keep their channels of elimination functioning well, and they use the yoga postures and deep breathing exercises of *hatha yoga* to develop suppleness and breath control.

You may need to work on your body if it is stiff and out of condition, through yoga, or any other form of exercise you enjoy

– whether swimming, dancing, or going to the gym.

You also need to clean up your diet if you have been overloading it with toxic foods. A liver cleansing diet for a fortnight is a good place to start, which avoids all alcohol, tea, coffee and stimulants, as well as sugar, fat, meat, dairy products, eggs and oranges. Sticking to a vegetable and rice-based diet after this will suit most body types.

As well as cleansing and detoxifying the body, it is important to purify the mind, which you can do with basic exercises.

The following exercises help to prepare you for Tantra, especially if you're not familiar with any kind of meditation practices. Meditation or yoga are excellent ways of preparing yourself for Tantra. Both these techniques help you to centre yourself, focusing inwards, rather than keeping your attention on the outside world.

CENTRING YOURSELF

This is a simple exercise, aimed at focusing your attention inward. It does this by training your attention to follow your breath, rather than being distracted by what's going on around you, or the thoughts chattering in your head. It introduces you to the central tantric technique of watching your breath, and imagining it moving up and down your back - following the main energy channel in your body.

- Stand with your feet hip distance apart, and your knees slightly bent, with your back straight. This helps align your spine so that energies can move more easily up and down your spine. Alternatively, you can sit on a chair with your feet on the ground, or sit in the yoga posture known as the tailor position, with your knees bent touching the floor, and the soles of your feet touching. It doesn't particularly matter whether you stand or sit, so long as your back is straight to enable the enery to move easily. Another alternative is the open lotus position, which is similar to the tailor position, but with the feet placed loosely one in front of the other, rather than touching.

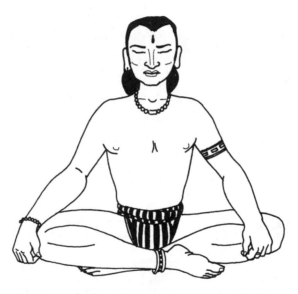

- Close your eyes and take a few minutes to go inside, focusing on your breathing. Focus on your inhalation and exhalation, and just allow your breathing to be as it is. You don't need to do anything apart from observe it. Notice that your breathing calms down and becomes longer and more even the longer you concentrate on it. As you inhale, imagine your breath is travelling down to the base of your spine, to your tailbone, or to the bones on which you are sitting. As you exhale, imagine it moving back up your spine to go out through your lungs. You can continue this for as long as you like – try to spend several minutes at least.

MEDITATION

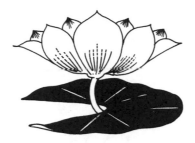

Internal worship purifies the mind. Purity of mind intensifies concentration and meditation. When meditation is ripe, enlightenment follows, and the seeker realizes the highest bliss.

Meditation practices have always played a large part in Tantric rituals. Before rushing into sexual practices, it is important to cultivate a meditative state of mind. Meditation is aimed at stilling our minds, in order to allow another dimension of experience to absorb us. As New Age writer Deepak Chopra says, to meditate doesn't mean you have to be doing anything special. You don't have to be sitting in advanced yoga postures, or chanting sacred sounds. What's important is that you take some time out every day, where you just sit quietly and allow your mind to switch off. All the techniques used by meditators, whether breathing, humming, chanting, or shaking the body, are designed to turn off the intrusive chattering of the mind, and make space for a different quality of experience. Chopra says you can just sit in a quiet room, in a comfortable armchair, gazing out the window, or listening to birdsong. If your mind can switch off while you're doing this, that's fine.

For many of us, however, it's difficult to stop intrusive thoughts coming in, perhaps evaluating what we're hearing or seeing, or thoughts about all the things we have to or want to do later on. Focusing the mind, by focusing attention on your breathing is the fundamental way that yogis begin to purify themselves for more advanced breathing techniques.

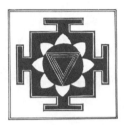

It is important to establish a regular meditation practice of some sort. It doesn't matter what form this takes. Some people can just sit quietly for 20 minutes, gazing without their mind wandering. Others use mantras (chants), or yantras to gaze at, to focus the mind on a still point of consciousness, calibrating the mind to spiritual forces around us. Traditional Tantric meditations often involve the imagery of fire – to burn away distractions and obstructions in the energy body.

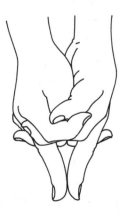

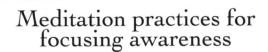

Meditation practices for focusing awareness

These instructions come from an ancient Tantric text, the *Vijnana Bhaivara*, thought to date from around the 6th century BC:

- Wherever your attention lights, experience without attachment.

- See *as if for the first time* an ordinary thing, with the consciousness of Shiva.

- Look at the empty space inside a bowl without seeing its walls. Be *absorbed* into this space, which is existence.

- Simply by looking steadily at the blue sky beyond the clouds, experience *divinity*.

- Intone a sound, such as a-u-m, slowly, hear the *sound of existence*.

- Be *absorbed* in the sound of a stringed instrument, or a song.

- When eating or drinking, become the taste of food and drink, and savour the *joy*.

- Wherever satisfaction is found, enter it deeply, and find *bliss*.

- At the start of sneezing, during fright or anxiety, feeling curious, at the beginning or end of hunger, experience profound *awareness*.

- Beloved, put attention neither on pleasure nor suffering, but in the place *between* these.

- Withdraw your mind from the object of desire and identify with desire. Then you *are* desire.

- Feel yourself *emanating* in all directions, which is your essential self.

- Eyes closed, see your inner being in detail. *See* your nature, which is divine.

- Place your whole attention on the energy channel, delicate as a lotus stem, in the centre of your spinal column. See the lightning-like Kundalini successively piercing each centre of energy. In this place, *be transformed*.

- Meditate on the *Shakti energy rising* from the muladhara chakra (at the base of the spine) like the rays of the sun, getting subtler and subtler until it dissolves into consciousness.

- Meditate on your body as *burning into ashes*, and become purified.

- During sexual union, *merge* into your beloved, and absorb the divine energy.

CREATING SACRED SPACE

Creating a sacred space means creating the kind of environment in which you can be relaxed, spontaneous and playful, as well as connected and still. Each object you bring into the sacred space can have its own meaning and associations for you. For instance, flowers bring in the element of beauty, while water can evoke fluidity.

- Clean the room – whether bedroom or an area of your living space – and clear it, getting rid of any unnecessary furniture, ornaments, magazines and clutter.

- Decorate the space with pictures, photographs or fabrics that create a relaxed and sensual mood.

- Ornament the room with flowers or sculpted objects like stones, shells, statues, etc.

- Music can be very helpful in creating a mood ambience. You'll need different pieces of music for different moods (see Resources section).

- Lighting needs to be soft and indirect. You can drape a shawl over a sidelight – or just use candles.

- Clothing should be soft and sensual; try a silky housecoat, kimono or a piece of printed fabric like a sarong.

- Scent the space with essential oils extracted from plants that soothe the nervous system and enhance erotic feelings. You can try ylang-ylang, gardenia, rose or another oil you like.

Tristan, 35: I've covered everything utilitarian in my bed-room with beautiful tapestries, which I've draped over shelves to form an altar space along one side of the room. There are floating candles in water all along the altar and around the room – I don't use an overhead light any more. On the altar I have an exquisite statue of Quan-yin, Chinese goddess of compassion, surrounded by lovely objects I've picked up over the years. I have an incense burner and different incenses for creating different moods. I keep some copper trays to hand, which I can use for food and drinks, or to make impromptu offerings to my partner. Our bed is on the floor, and I've covered the carpets with oriental rugs and scatter cushions, so that wherever we are we feel cosy and enclosed.

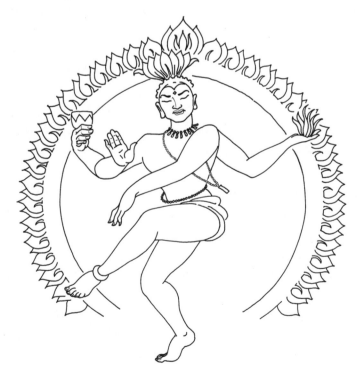

CREATING A TANTRIC BED

A Tantric bed is a sensual haven rather than a prosaic space for sleeping in.

The aesthetic quality of your bed can be enhanced with thin muslin drapes, or silk hangings. The quality of your linens and coverings can be sensuous, with textures and sensations that seduce your skin. Typical Tantric colours are red, yellow and orange. Cushions are good for comfort while exploring each others bodies, or taking Tantric postures.

You will need your accoutrements to hand – feathers, essential oils, and perhaps some inspirational paintings of lovers, or an Indian or Tibetan statue of the divine couple in embrace.

Ariane, 38: My fantasy Tantric bed is made of soft velvet cushions, crimson, purple, lilac, tasselled and jewelled. A vast haven marooned in space. Soft mattress, overblown. The mattress is full of duck feathers, a fine silk veil shimmers in the breeze. The French windows are surrounded by jasmine and hibiscus, and open onto a private courtyard with a water fountain raining gently over the lotus pond. Koi flirt with the sun and shade, or bask upside down in gentle arcs. The room is scented with open flowers, and scented oils are arrayed at the bedside. Peacock feathers, ostrich plumes, delicate fluff are in reach on a tray. On the little altar Tantric idols bless us; gods in priapic stance, consorting with ecstatic goddesses; the virgin looks on benevolently, glassy tears glisten on her snowy maternal cheeks. An Egyptian mummy stands guard.

CREATING RITUAL SPACE

Pip, 46: My partner and I tried to follow a book about Tantra. We failed miserably and usually ended up arguing. If you've not experienced the special energy of practising Tantra it seems either stupid or impossible to pretend that you are a god or a goddess. If you've not experienced the Tantric space, which is one of altered consciousness, you feel false, artificial, as if you're just fooling around. Some people seem to 'get it' straight from the book, but most of us seem to need help in being initiated into the particular energy of Tantra. Then you can go back to the book because then you understand what it's all about on a feeling level.

Tantric space is deliberately created in both a physical sense and an energetic sense. When running Tantric groups, workshop leaders turn the room into a temple of love, and create an altar on which they deliberately place objects of beauty and symbolism in such a way as to evoke the spirits of Shakti and Shiva. You can create your own altar to the principles of Shakti and Shiva with objects representing the qualities of the goddess and god, which embody the divine. Ritual is what transforms the workshop experience from a therapy style of experience into something more spiritual.

Martin, 45: I've made an altar in my bedroom. There's a photo of my Tibetan teacher, and a Shri yantra on the wall behind. I have male objects on the right side – some Tibetan double cymbals and a Buddha – and female objects on the left – a statue of the goddess Tara and a bell. Each of the five elements are represented: a glass of water, a crystal for earth, candles for fire, a feather for air, and a stick of incense which reminds me of space as I watch the smoke curling upwards. It feels magical when the candles and incense are lit, and just the act of lighting them quietens my mind. In daily life I tend to get speedy and distracted, but the habitual action of lighting the candles helps me to change pace.

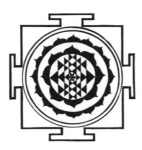

Ritual is about inviting, or allowing the sacred into our lives. Ritual space is about having an intention to do things in a particular atmosphere. We can create a ritual space through association. The processes of clearing up clutter in the room, covering up any work things, and taking off the telephone so it won't intrude are all part of clearing your own psychic space of mundane distractions. If we learn to associate activities like lighting candles and incense, and greeting each other with the Hindu form of greeting, a *namaste,* with Tantric ritual, then just doing these things will put us into a Tantric frame of mind.

Ritual helps us to create the atmosphere we need to do things with a sense of sacredness. It is this sense of sacredness that can help us step beyond our normal limits, into closer connection with our partners, and into a much more intense sexual experience. The sexual exercises are not just about appetising sex, they're about sacred sex. This means that sexual exchange should take place in ritual space.

In all ritual, having the right intention is crucial. Intention just means holding a thought with a particular purpose in mind. Because your energy follows your thoughts, creating a clear intention means that your energy will flow in the direction you want it to. If you're not sure what you're doing and why, your energy will move in an unclear way. If you are thinking clearly, then the divine energies you're calling on can move clearly through a clear conduit. In traditional Tantra, meditating on yantras, and chanting lots of mantras is used as a way of focusing the mind and creating the right intention.

CREATING THE TANTRIC FIELD

The most essential aspect of ritual is doing things with awareness. It is having the quality of being present with what you are doing, or what you would like to happen once you've finished preparing the space, without your mind running on other things.

Important elements that help to create the ambience of ritual are candles (or flame), water and smells. You can choose to include the five elements in your sacred space by setting out a bowl of water, perhaps with a flower floating in it, a candle (fire), a saucer of salt (earth), a feather (air) and incense (for space).

- If you want to make your own yantra for ritual use, you can use rice, sand or any other material to trace the design on the floor, or on large sheets of paper. The physical act of making the design helps create an appropriate internal attitude.

- You can mark the sacred space out by sounding a gong, or any sort of drum. Some people use singing bowls, which produce a lovely ringing sound.

- The mantra *om* can be used at the beginning and end of your time together to open and close the ritual space. Hindu yogis regard *om* as the primordial sound of the universe, and reciting it helps to harmonize us with the energy of the cosmos.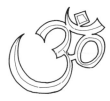

- Music is helpful to create and sustain a certain mood, and a particular association to that mood. Calm relaxing music is best, and it's nice to have it playing on an endless loop if you don't want to break the atmosphere by changing tapes (see Resources).

Julie, 34: My partner and I went to the beach and collected 17 large white stones washed by the stream. After lighting a stick of incense and candle at the altar, and invoking the goddess Tara through singing her mantra, we laid the stones in a circle around the room taking turns, using each stone laying as an opportunity to banish negative feelings that often creep into our relationship, and to call in the positive, affirming qualities we felt we needed. This created a sense of safety, both physically because we felt enclosed in this special circle, and psychologically, because we had heard each other name the qualities each of us wanted to invoke or banish.

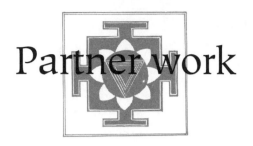

Partner work

HONOURING YOUR PARTNER: NAMASTE

Start each ritual with a *namaste* – the Hindu form of greeting. *Namaste* means 'I honour you as an aspect of myself,' or 'I honour you as an aspect of God.'

You will develop an association with the greeting, which will help you to create a Tantric approach with your partner – once you've overcome any feelings of foolishness.

- Stand 2–3 feet apart facing your partner, so you can bow to each other comfortably. Focus on your breathing for a few moments.

- Gaze into your partner's eyes. To help keep your eyes focused when you're close to each other, it can be better to gaze into your partner's left eye.

- As you breathe in, imagine drawing your energy up to your heart and bringing your palms together in front of your heart, in the gesture of prayer.

- As you breathe out, bring your foreheads together, shifting the focus of your gaze to the centre of your partner's eyebrows. Focus your awareness on the meeting of your third eye chakra.

- As you breathe in, draw your awareness back to your heart centre.

- As you breathe out allow your energy back down towards the earth, and allow your hands to come down to your sides.

CLEARING THE AIR

The Tantric attitude is to meet everything in an attitude of respect and reverence. In so doing, you honour your partner, and experience yourself as connected to the other. They are a mirror to you. In honouring your partner as an aspect of yourself, you automatically step into a heartful space of honouring and respecting the other, and taking responsibility for yourself and your own feelings.

If you haven't cleared yourself and centred yourself it's hard to start on any Tantric ritual. Anger and resentment will prevent any sort of enlightenment experience. You can't be fully present if you're stuck in past problems, or negative exchanges that took place between you. If there are negative emotions between you, you need to clear the air with a duo-logue, aimed at constructive conflict resolution. This duo-logue is similar to the basic marriage guidance technique of getting couples to clear the air. The Tantric spin on it is to conduct the duo-logue within sacred space, with the intention of getting beyond your inter-personal issues and connecting with the love between you.

- Bow to your partner: this helps you to open your heart towards your partner by acknowledging and appreciating them – even if they have angered or hurt you in some way. It doesn't work if you do this grudgingly. You are trying to connect with the core of your partner. All these feelings of hurt are to do with the ego (an over-developed sense of self-importance), and the ego taking offence at perceived threats to the self.

  The *namaste* signals your intent to let go of whatever is standing between you. You create an intention to relate to the essence of your partner, and to re-connect with the love between you.

- Each person then has 5–7 minutes of pre-agreed time to talk without interruption, about whatever is on their mind, without blaming the other person. Remember to talk about your own feelings, rather than trying to tell the other person what is wrong with them, or blame them.

- Keep swapping over until there is nothing left to say.

- If you can't resolve an issue, you can agree a time to discuss it further. If you can't let go of the negative emotions you should leave your Tantric practice for another time. If you constantly get stuck, you will need outside help or counselling to help you find a way through your communication difficulties.

- Since most disagreement is about 5% content and 95% emotions (e.g. anger), another option is to just shout and scream at your partner in complete gibberish, meaningless, nonsense words. You can jump around and wave your arms around till the energy has dissipated – usually into laughter.

- Once you've cleansed yourself of negative emotions, you are more free to allow the flow of feelings into your experience.

In honouring our partner we step automatically into the heart space of honouring and respecting the other person, and taking responsibility for our actions. The idea is to become conscious of not projecting the shadow aspect we reject about ourselves onto the other person, making them into an enemy. If you are embracing all aspects of yourself, you don't need to project qualities outside. Traditional religious systems separate good from evil, forcing people to create external enemy figures. In Tantra we heal this split by accepting what's good AND bad about ourselves.

CONNECTING

Adrian 43: I find that I lose energy when I start over analyzing the relationship. The more we talk, the more the energy between us seems to diminish.

What is wonderful when we connect properly is to feel so completely in the body. Your mind is at a complete standstill. Words are just to facilitate the here and now – to enhance whatever's happening between us, and strengthen the connection. They're just to do with what is happening at that particular moment – nothing else.

Whenever you're having a discussion all your past and your history comes up, as well as your fears for the future. All these things just destroy the relationship. You get the same old familiar feeling of going round in circles, talking without making any progress.

When we get caught up in analyzing what's going on between us, the expression in my partner's eyes changes so quickly. From caring, concern and openness, and a sense of focus, all that is lost and it feels like we're not in contact anymore.

Connecting is as important, or even more important than actually doing anything. Once you've connected properly, you're more than halfway there in terms of being in a Tantric space. Tantric sex is not about routinely doing any of the suggested exercises, or getting into fancy positions, it's about introducing a different quality of awareness into your love-making.

Tuning in to yourself and your partner involves emptying out the cup – clearing the air of any emotional stuff that's hanging between you. Getting rid of emotional stuff in order to allow something magical to happen. If you try to create something through force of will, or one partner is trying to make the other partner do something, it will all backfire. The essence of it is to connect, and then see what the energy of the two of you together allows in. At least half of the time you spend on Tantric ritual should be spent preparing and connecting, the rest actually doing something together.

SEEING YOUR PARTNER AS AN ENERGY BODY

Eye gazing

The aim of this exercise is to create a soul connection through looking deeply into the eyes of your beloved. The eyes are considered the windows to the soul.

- Sitting on the floor in open lotus posture with your back straight, legs opened out, bent at the knee with your feet loosely one in front of the other, gaze into your partner's eyes. Don't sit so close that you become cross-eyed: you need to be able to hold your partner's gaze comfortably, for some time.

- Hold each other's gaze steadily, without letting your eyes flick all over their face, or wander off around the room. Just look and observe your partner, your Beloved. Gaze at them without thoughts, without assessing their appearance or anything about them. Try to settle your mind, and just be in the presence of your Beloved.

- Without speaking, look *into* your Beloved. Open your heart to your Beloved.

- Synchronize your breath. In Tantric exercises the man usually follows the pace of the woman's breathing. (You can swap over later.)

- While looking into your partner's eyes, focus on the sacred connection between the two of you, and then gradually extend your awareness out into the whole world, feeling a connection with the universe.

Spoon

This is a relaxing exercise to do with your partner to connect before making love, or as part of love-making, or before going off to sleep.

- Lie on your left side, with one person's back to your partner's abdomen. It doesn't matter who is on the outside and who on the inside, but you should both be lying on your left side. This aligns up the energetic centres or chakras.

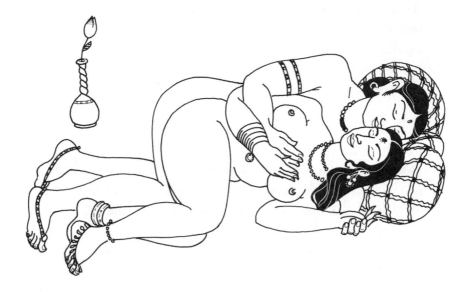

- Concentrate on your breath as it passes in and out of your nostrils.
  Then become aware of your partner's breath. Harmonize your
  breathing with your partner's. The person at the back follows the
  pace of the person at the front.

- Breathe in together, hold, then breathe out together. Pause before
  breathing in again.

- The person lying behind their partner imagines that with every exhalation they send the energy of their breath into the heart centre in
  their partner's subtle body.

- Once your breath is synchronized, start working on visualizing your
  chakras at the same time. You can use a colour or the symbol for each
  chakra to help you tune in. One partner can call out the name of the
  chakra so the other can meet them in the same place.

- Together, starting with your base chakras, imagine you're breathing in and out together from this centre. After four or five breaths, move up to the next chakra.

- Continue the process until you reach your crown chakra, at the very top of your head.

TUNING IN

Opening your heart: devotion

The term puja traditionally refers to devotional rituals dedicated to the goddess and gods. In Tantra you worship your Beloved as the other half of yourself. In worshipping them, you are worshipping divinity and yourself as divinity. The ceremonial components of puja include invocation, welcoming, seating, washing the feet, offering water, flowers and perfumes, and dainties like honey or sweetmeats, lighting candles and incense, and prayer or meditation. These rituals are all commonplace at temples throughout the world, and are important means of creating an internal feeling of devotion. You can use any or all of these rituals to worship your partner, if you wish to. Traditionally puja involved cleaning the body, and the temple space; washing the temple with fresh water, scattering rose petals, leaving offerings of food. Bathing is always helpful as it relaxes both the receiver and giver. Traditional Tantric practitioners would ritually wash the different parts of their body, including the mouth and nose. We tend to shower, which of course washes all parts of the body at the same time. All we need to be aware of is washing our body with attention and love – or better still, washing your lover's body with loving devotion.

The most important gift you can give to your partner is a sense of loving devotion.

To invoke the divine in your partner, worship them as the embodiment of the divine. Treat them as the god or goddess they really are. Try and keep this element of devotional worship alive as you interact with your partner. You don't need to be overly serious, but you do need to make them feel appreciated, and as if you really feel they are divine.

Really look at your partner, lovingly, whenever you are engaged in something together. That helps your partner feel really seen, and cared for. Deepak Chopra says 'the only true need anyone has is to be seen as real.' If your eyes are slipping away, or onto objects around the room, it is hard for your partner to feel there's a safe level of intimacy or that you're really seeing them. Whenever you feel your attention wandering off on endless thoughts and distractions, bring yourself right back to the present moment with your partner. It's helpful to be in a quiet space with tranquil music, candle light, comfortable cushions – whatever

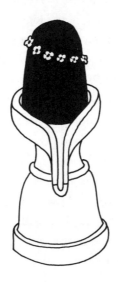

makes you both relax and feel safe. Allow yourself enough time and do not hurry through the process of acknowledging and worshipping your partner. Remember there is no goal to hurry towards – only the pleasure of the journey.

Yin-yang game

Ariane, 38: My partner and I played this game over a whole weekend. He wanted me to build a fire for him on the beach, so I collected a mound of driftwood. At first his mood was one of revelling in the sudden permission to determine exactly how everything was to be. He gave me orders in an offensive manner, but according to the rules of the game I swallowed my habitual retorts and humoured his whims. As he sat on the beach, watching the firewood gather as the sun went down over the fishing boats, his mood softened. He started to build the fire he'd long wanted to have on this beach, and we both dropped into a calm, tranquil feeling, like meditation but without doing anything. Focusing on the fire, we started some fire breathing, sitting in yab-yom together (with me on his lap) and my big cloak draped around us. This led spontaneously to riding the wave of bliss together, in which we dissolved into each other. It was no longer his desires I was meeting, but the two of us merged into desire.

In this game, one of you is active (yang), asking for your wishes to be met, while the other does all she or he can to meet those needs. This doesn't involve doing anything you don't want to do. It's not a power trip. The aim is to encourage the active person to voice their own thoughts and desires, rather than worrying about

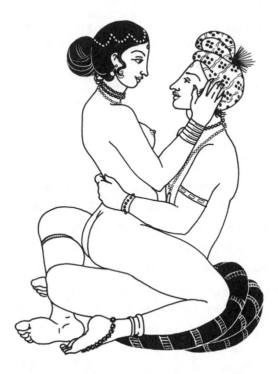

whether whatever they're doing is pleasing their partner or not. It is about learning to receive, without having to give at the same time. You can use this game to explore non-sexual desires, as well as sexual or sensual experiences. You may want to be massaged, or cooked for, or taken out. Or you may want to direct your partner in making love to you.

The structure is very simple. You agree a period of time, anything from 30 minutes to a whole day. For that time you determine the activities you would like you both to do. You can ask for what you want, and how you would like it to be. You can give your partner feedback about the way they are fulfilling your needs.

The yin (receptive) person tries to remain tuned in and sensitive to the needs of their partner, focusing on giving and encouraging their partner to explore their desires. As always in Tantra, it's not necessary to do anything you don't want to do. If you feel your partner is asking for something that makes you uncomfortable, just tell him or her gently that you're sorry, you can't fulfil that particular request right now, but you'd be happy to do something else.

Ask what else they would like you to do for or with them.

Nancy, 33: I get stubborn when my partner asks me to do something. I feel put upon and I don't want to oblige. I resent being told what to do. Either I feel subjugated because I hate having my leadership taken away, or I feel deflated, as if I'm doing the wrong thing and then I withdraw. The next morning my partner says 'Hey, what happened? You disappeared on me.'

The best way to get rid of these feelings is for us to go out all night dancing, just clearing away all that negativity.

I can always find reasons not to make love – like having to get up early in the morning. But Tantra counteracts this by reiterating the importance of connecting. It helps keep channels of communication open and we've become more emotionally supportive.

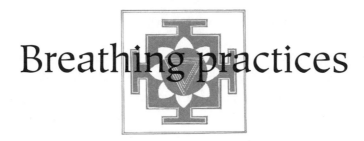

Breathing practices

The more advanced or complicated exercises are not necessarily the most intimate ones, or the most powerful ones.

Tina, 36: One of the most challenging exercises I did was the synchronised breathing. I sat with my legs out with my partner sitting on my lap. I tried to breathe her breath in through my genitals and then breathe out into her mouth. We just couldn't co-ordinate our in and out breath and we got really frustrated. Not quite getting it right highlighted lots of issues in our relationship. Neither of us is brilliant at communicating, and instead of stopping struggling and discussing it we just went silent on each other.

But afterwards we did say how hard it was, and asked ourselves why we didn't just stop and sort it out. Just discussing it brought us closer together again, and next time we tried it, we were able to do the exercise.

Doing these exercises keeps pushing me, and challenging me. I always learn a lot when the exercises are difficult. There's a part of me that doesn't trust, and doesn't know how to let go. I hate being led in exercises where we're playing at leading or being led. That's an issue in our relationship. I want to let go of control and it really frustrates me when I can't. In the past I had to be always sexually active, now I'm getting better at lying back, and receiving.

These exercises put a torchlight on relationship patterns;

ours are mainly around communication. They help me be more aware, and I'm working on my blocks.

COMPLETE BREATHING

The aim of this exercise is to learn to breath fully, right down into your abdomen. It enables you to open your lungs more when breathing, and slow down the rate of your breathing. These are the first steps to developing more complex breathing exercises for use in Tantric sex.

There are four parts to traditional yogic breathing:

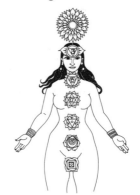

- a slow inhalation

- holding the breath for several seconds (once this becomes comfortable)

- a slow exhalation

- then a pause before the next inhalation.

This is called the complete breath, because the pause allows your awareness to expand out beyond the process of breathing. Practice the complete breath until it feels easy and natural, starting with only a short pause after inhalation and exhalation.

Once you are comfortable with this breath, you can begin to visualize the breath flowing in through your lungs and down your central energetic channel, which contemporary Tantric teachers call the inner flute. Take the breath right down to the base chakra, at the base of your spine, and then allow your breath to flow up again, passing through the heart centre on the way.

Tantric breath is concerned with balancing and uniting the upward and downward breath (which symbolize energy and consciousness). You can imagine inhaling air as if it were a fluid, lighter than water. While holding the breath in, visualize yourself absorbing the vitality of the air in your lungs. While breathing out you can imagine that your breath is a fire which burns up all impurities.

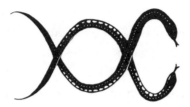

Solar-lunar breath

The aim of this exercise is to balance your breath, using alternate nostril breathing. The rhythm of your breath is roughly even, equal between breathing in, holding, and breathing out:

- Sit in the open lotus position, or with crossed legs, back and head straight.

- First bend the index and middle fingers of your right hand into the palm, and use your right thumb to close your right nostril. Inhale through the left nostril, focusing your mind on the air gently flowing into your lungs. Concentrate on the vital energy you are inhaling along with the air.

- Once you have inhaled fully, hold your breath while closing both nostrils between your thumb and ring finger. Hold in your breath for a count of four, if this feels comfortable.

- Then lift your thumb up, while you exhale through your right nostril, keeping the left nostril closed with the ring finger. Inhale again, focusing on all the energy you're breathing in.

• Again press both nostrils closed to retain your breath.

Once you exhale through your left nostril, by lifting your ring finger, you've done one whole round of Solar-Lunar breathing. Try starting with five to ten rounds of breathing.

This technique consciously unites your solar and lunar breaths. When these are in balance, the life-force can travel up the *sushumna* channel at the axis of the body, the inner flute. If you find this technique easy, or intriguing, you can try it out with your partner during lovemaking.

Yogis believe that lying on one side causes the opposite side's nostril to dominate the breathing pattern. The Tantras suggest that the man consciously draws in the exhaled air from the woman's left nostril through his right nostril, and allow her to consciously breathe in his exhaled breath from the right nostril through her left nostril. Face-to-face lovemaking with each partner lying on his/her side facilitates this exchange naturally.

Be conscious of the breath during lovemaking and focus on the exchange of vital energy that happens as you exchange breaths.

HEART TO HEART BREATHING

The aim of this exercise is to focus your breathing on your heart chakra, connecting your own heart chakra with that of your partner. When you inhale, draw your breath down from your mouth, into your heart area.

Practise the exercise alone first. It will help you to go inside fully, and not get distracted about what your partner is doing, or trying to synchronize the process with your partner.

You can practise this exercise standing, sitting with a straight spine, or lying on your back with your knees bent:

- Close your eyes with your hands on your heart. This helps you to focus on sending the energy to that area.

- As you breathe in, draw the energy into your heart.

- Pause at the end of the in-breath, focusing on your heart area.

- Release your breath, and allow it to slowly exhale.

- Continue this heart breath for several minutes.

- You may want to use some soft, heartful music as an accompaniment to the breathing.

Once you feel comfortable with the heart breath, and it becomes easy to increase the awareness in your heart area, you are ready to work with your partner. Start with bowing to each other. It's best to do this exercise with eyes open, gazing at each other throughout. You can allow your feelings of loving heartfullness to be expressed through your eyes, as well as through the energy connection you're creating with your breath.

If you lose your concentration, or start to feel self-conscious, just close your eyes and concentrate on following your own breathing pattern, as you did when you were alone:

- Stand facing each other, and gaze into each other's eyes.

- Place your right hand (giving hand) on your partner's heart, as you are both giving your heart energy to each other.

- With your out-breath imagine breathing the energy from your heart into their heart.

- With your in-breath imagine inhaling their heart energy into your heart.

- Once you feel comfortable with this, try breathing alternately; you breathe in as your partner breathes out. As you breathe out, they then breathe in. The breath becomes a vehicle for the heart energy to be exchanged between you. You breath the loving energy in as they send it to you from their heart, then you send them your loving energy through your breath.

- You can practise swapping over hands later on.

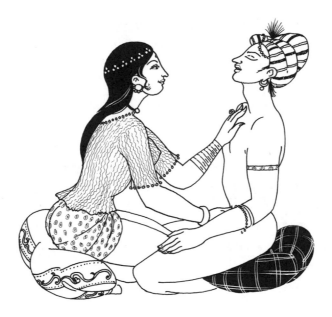

SEX AND THE HEART BREATH

This exercise should be practised alone at first, to get used to visualizing your breath arising from your base chakra.

In this exercise you start to use the Tantric technique of imagining your breath climbing through the chakras in your body. When you inhale, you don't imagine that your breath is going down from your mouth, into your lungs and heart. Instead, you imagine that you are inhaling your breath through your genitals, and as you breathe in, drawing it up from your genitals through the centre of your body, and into the area of your heart.

This exercise should be practised alone at first, to get used to visualizing your breath arising from your base chakra.

- Place one hand on your heart and the other on your sex. Imagine that you are breathing in through your yoni (or your imaginary yoni if you are a man).

- Feel your breath drawing energy up through your sex. Breathe up from your genitals, drawing the energy up the centre of your body and into your heart by the end of each in-breath.

- Pause at the end of the in-breath, focusing your awareness on your heart area.

- Release your breath, and allow it to drop down again, through the centre of your body, or your spine, down to the tailbone and your genital area.

- Then practise the exercise with your partner, breathing at the same time together. Start with a namaste greeting.

- Stand or sit in an open lotus posture facing each other, and gaze into each other's eyes.

- You both inhale at the same time, imagining you are drawing your breath up through your genitals, into your heart area.

- Then exhale together, imagining your breath receding from your heart area into your sex, and out through the base of your spine.

It can be helpful to use your right hand to gesture that the energy is coming up from your sex into your heart. At the end of the in-breath, as you pause, you can complete the gesture in an offering to your partner (just in front of your heart area). The gesture is as if you were offering a beautiful flower, or a lotus to them. It is in the area of your heart that the energy of both of you is coming together. As your breath falls again, your hand can follow its pathway down the front of your body back to your sex. This can be helpful to you both in feeling co-ordinated, as you can see the path of the breath by watching the rhythm of the hand rising and falling.

You can extend this exercise by taking the breath up to the higher chakras to connect sex with heart and then with spirit. Follow the steps of the heart wave, bringing your energy from your sex up to your heart for several minutes, creating a strong heart connection before going further with the exercise. Then bring the energy up to the third eye.

Using your hand to gesture will help your partner know when you are moving up from the heart chakra. The woman (shakti) will decide this changeover by letting the breath drop down into her sex, and then taking the next breath right up into the third eye chakra – the energy centre located on your forehead between your eyes.

It is particularly helpful to stay in eye contact with your partner. It helps you have a sense of the vision you share of uniting sexuality and spirituality.

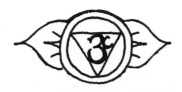

HEART WAVE

In the heart wave you create an energy connection between you and your beloved, in which you share your loving, sexual energy at the level of your heart and sex.

This exercise should be practised with your partner:

Once you feel comfortable with the previous exercise, try developing it so that you are breathing alternately; you breathe in as your partner breathes out. As you breathe out, your partner breathes in. The breath becomes a vehicle for the heart energy to be connected between you.

You can start with breathing together and later switch to alternate breathe. If you start with breathing together, you can focus on drawing your breath up through your genitals and into your heart, offering it to your partner during the pause in your breath, and then letting it drop back down again on the exhalation.

To change over to alternate breathing, the woman (Shakti) holds her breath in the heart chakra while her partner (Shiva) breathes out. Then as he begins to inhale, she releases her breath, visualizing her energy dropping back down to her sex. It may help to imagine yourself as swinging your energy in a crescent shape between sex and heart – these are the points at which your own energy is connecting with that of your partner.

It can be tricky to co-ordinate this alternate breath, but it's very important for later exercises which use the breath to circulate energy between you.

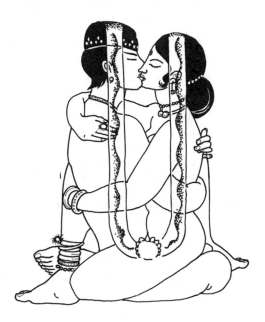

Nancy, 33: There are times when my breath is in rhythm, when I breathe in my partner's breath as she breathes out. After a few minutes I feel like the boundaries between us are breaking up. I lose the sense of my own edges, and my separateness from her.

It helps us to get out of our heads, and creates a feeling of intimacy. We both tend to keep a bit of ourselves back, even when our bodies are there – it's like saying "See, you haven't got all of me".

This is a good way for us to connect. The energy is being circulated and a sexual charge starts to build up between us. Sometimes we forget to breathe when we're excited, especially when my partner tenses up and holds back from an orgasm. So we remind each other to breathe. Whenever we get stuck with something, we go back to simply breathing. Whenever we're getting aroused but there's a feeling of holding back, breathing and moving around a bit can help.

Because we tend to have different arrival times sexually, breathing together helps me keep a sense of what my partner is experiencing.

MALE AND FEMALE BREATH

The aim of this is to build energy and to harmonise the energies between the two of you as a couple. The 'male breath' is associated with giving, and the 'female breath' is associated with receiving. In playing with this breath, and swapping roles during the exercise, you can play with alternating giving and receiving. This exercise helps to balance and circulate your breathing as a couple, and helps you explore different energetic qualities as you alternate breathing.

The basic technique is to breathe in through your genitals, and out through your heart. Women breathe in through their yonis. For men, the area of their imaginary yoni is in the perineum. The 'male' breath is out through the genitals, and in through the heart. The 'female' breath is out through the heart and in through the genitals. Practise both forms of breathing alone first of all, and then with your partner.

Sit in open lotus position facing each other. If you want a sense of greater connection and closeness, sit in yab-yom (illustrated on page 140), where the man sits in an open lotus position and the woman sits on the man's lap and wraps her legs around his waist. The man needs to be very comfortable on cushions, with hips and thighs supported to carry the weight of his partner:

- Start your practice with Shakti (the woman) breathing in through the genitals and out through the heart, sending this heart energy to her partner. Imagine breathing the energy from your heart into their heart.

- As the woman breathes out, Shiva (the man) breathes in through his heart, absorbing her loving energy. He should imagine inhaling her heart energy into his heart, drawing it down into his genitals as she exhales, releasing erotic love through the genitals.

- The woman then breathes in, breathing the erotic energy she receives though his genitals, into her yoni, and drawing it up to her heart area.

- This creates a delicious circling of loving and erotic energy between the two energy systems of the couple. Try changing the direction of the energy circle, so that the woman is doing the 'male breath', sending her erotic energy out through her yoni, into her partner's lingam, which the man then takes into his heart centre, transforming into heartful loving energy which he directs to the heart centre of his beloved.

- Explore both the male and female breath. The male breath is not reserved for men, rather this describes who is being more active in the breath and energy transfer. The female breath is considered more receptive. Depending on whether you are playing with your outer

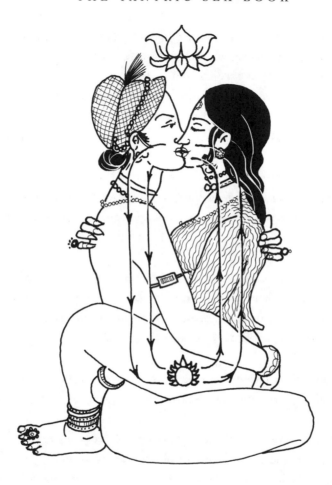

female, or your inner male energies, one or the other will feel more comfortable.

- Notice which modality (male or female), and which pole (heart or sex) feels most comfortable. (This will change according to your own internal state, and the dynamics of your relationship).

- Explore different paces of breathing; faster, slower, more intense. In setting the pace of the breath it is usually Shakti who leads, although you can of course re-negotiate this. The aim is to find your own rhythm and learn how to harmonize your rhythm with your partner's.

Once you've become familiar with this exercise, and the energies it arouses and moves around your body, you may want to physically connect your genitals, to intensify the sense of connectedness and increase the erotic charge. This will give you a taste of sacred sex, in which your physical and energetic bodies are connected, and your sexual connection transformed through your loving connection.

Once you're both feeling sexually aroused by the breathing and circulating of energy, you can continue the breathing with your genitals connected. In Tantra this transition occurs at the woman's instigation, since she is Shakti. If she feels she would like her partner to enter her, she invites his lingam inside her yoni, or takes his lingam inside her as she sits on his lap in yabyom. This is the best posture to hold while doing this exercise, whether the genitals are physically connected or not.

Ariane, 38: I was having trouble synchronizing my breathing with that of my partner. I felt he was always breathing too fast for me, which meant that we either got out of synch with our breathing, or I started hyperventilating. I preferred a slower, more meditative style of breathing, rather than one that made me feel like he was getting more and more aroused, and running on ahead of me.

At the same time I felt he was always hassling me to have intercourse, rather than taking time over love-making and not being in such a rush to be inside me. We decided to have an individual session with our Tantric teacher, who asked us to show him how we did the male-female breath. He immediately noticed that I was very uncomfortable with my partner doing the male breath, feeling his sexual energy as intrusive, and he suggested that for a period of time we just worked on my leading with the male breath and him using the female breath, so that he could become more receptive to my sexual energy.

SYNCHRONIZED BREATHING

The aim of this exercise is to synchronize your breathing, using visualization to raise the energy from your base chakra through your higher chakras, together as a couple.

Once you become familiar with the visualization you can add some gentle pelvic rocking, to open up and charge the energy in your pelvis. If you suffer from a stiff pelvis it can be helpful to do some warm up exercises first to loosen the hips and pelvis.

These movements come from oriental dancing, and feel very natural to the body. While standing, with knees slightly bent, practise tracing circles with your hips, as if you were dancing with a hula hoop – but slowly. Then trace figures of eight, both horizontally and vertically.

- Sit facing each other, at first in the open lotus position. Later you can move into the yab-yom position, in which the woman sits on the man's lap with her legs wrapped around his waist. If Shakti is too heavy for Shiva, she can place a cushion under her buttocks to help support her. In either position, you can gaze into each other's eyes.

- Breathe slowly and gently, falling into a slow, deep rhythm. The woman sets the pace of this breathing, but should adjust if her partner's pace is

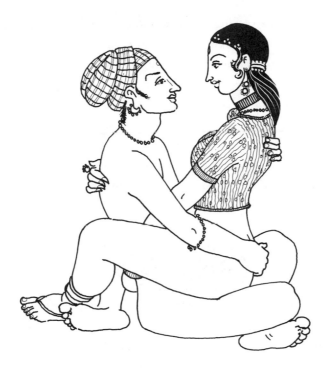

very different from hers. As the breathing establishes a natural rhythm, you can both close your eyes and focus on the visualizations and internal work.

- Start drawing the breath up through the base of your spine. As you breathe in, draw the energy up into your first chakra and as you exhale let it go back out through to the base of your spine (around your perineum).

- Once you have established this pattern, introduce a gentle tilting of the pelvis, forward (with genitals facing downwards) as you breathe in, and then tilting backwards (with genitals facing towards each other), as you breathe in.

- Continue with the rocking of the pelvis, both of you bringing your energy up to the second chakra. As you breathe in bring your hips forward, as you breathe out, tilt your hips backwards.

- Continue this exercise going through each of the chakras in turn, gently rocking with each breath. You can follow the movement of energy through your chakras, and as it reaches the heart chakra make a gesture with your hand of offering this energy to your partner. This helps you both to do this at the same time, together.

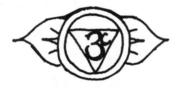

- Draw the breath up to the third eye centre and offer it to each other, together. As usual, the woman leads this changeover.

- Once you're familiar with this exercise, you can add on an extra stage, drawing the energy up to the crown centre together.

ALTERNATE BREATHING

This exercise is similar to the previous one, but breathing alternately enables you to circulate energy between you. It is similar to the male/female breath with the addition of pelvic rocking to build more erotic charge in your pelvis.

- Sit facing each other, at first in open lotus position (later you can move into yab-yom).

- The woman starts: draw your breath in through your yoni as you rock your pelvis and hips gently backwards (with yoni forwards).

- Visualize your breath climbing up to your heart, and, when you exhale, send your breath out through your heart into the heart of your lover. You may wish to use hand gestures to show him where your breath is located, drawing the breath from your genitals up the front of your body and offering it in an opening hand gesture at the level of your heart centre. (Keeping up the pelvis rocking with each inhalation and exhalation.)

- The man inhales your breath through his heart and sends it down through his energy channels and exhales out through his lingam. The woman inhales through her yoni as he exhales out through his genitals.

- After several cycles of circulating the energy between you, you will feel a growing sense of love and unity.

UNITY THROUGH SACRED SOUND

This is an exercise described by spiritual teacher Ram Dass, which combines mantras and breath, in which you circulate the power word *om* through the connection you have created between your two hearts. The aim is to experience your partner as an energetic mirror of yourself, and then merge into union with your partner.

- Both partners sit in a comfortable position facing each other. Gaze into each other's right eye. Find a rhythm of breathing together that is slow, deep, and trusting.

- Co-ordinate your breath so that you are breathing in as your partner is breathing out. Once co-ordination is established, visualize your breathing as the waves of the ocean, rolling in and out with each breath.

- After a short period, one partner begins to say, aloud, *om* with the out breath, directing the sound to the heart chakra of the other. As the first partner begins to breathe in again, the other one breathes out, chanting the *om* on the out breath.

- After several rounds of breathing you'll both feel a deepening of connection and completion. At the end you can rest in the awareness of oneness by closing your eyes. Keep up your co-ordinated breathing and humming.

Meditation and visualization

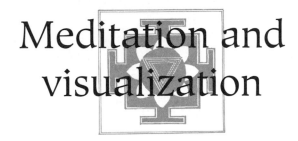

UNITING HEAVEN AND EARTH: MEDITATION

This meditation is geared towards connecting the red and white energies internally and unifying the solar and lunar elements. It uses it as a means of connecting the sensual world with the plane of spirit and of using the image of fire to purify your chakras. This meditation can be done on your own, or you can lead your partner through this guided meditation. You can put it on a cassette tape so that you can both follow it or you can get a tape recorded by Tantra teacher Leora Lightwoman (see Resources section):

- Sit in a comfortable position, either cross-legged on the floor, or sitting in a chair with your feet on the ground and your back straight. Imagine that you are growing roots down into the ground, from the base of your spine, if you are sitting cross-legged, or through the soles of your feet. Imagine these are energetic roots, reaching deep into the earth.

- As you breathe in and out, imagine these roots expanding, growing, reaching through the layers of earth and layers of rock, until you can start to sense the heat coming from the centre of the earth. With each out-breath allow your roots to go deeper and deeper – into the molten lava at the centre of the earth. Feel the intense heat, and imagine that through this heat you're contacting the hot, fiery core of the earth, symbolizing your connection to the life force, to life, to the material source of energy, and feel the energy this brings you. Your roots connecting you to this hot fiery core symbolizes your connectedness to this source of life.

- As you continue to breathe, draw up this heat and redness, this source of life and energy. It is your own passion, your lust for life, and your desire to be alive in this body, on this planet here and now. Keep breathing and drawing this energy up through your roots, right into the soles of your feet. Feel the heat, or imagine it's there, in the soles of your feet.

- Allow the warmth to permeate up your legs. Draw that red-hot energy into your pelvis, allowing it to burn away anything that is not aligned with your love of life, with joy, with vibrancy. Breathe in, drawing that heat into your abdomen. Imagine it burning away any obstacles to your being fully in your passion, in your vitality.

- Then draw that energy into your lungs and chest, allowing your lungs to expand with the fullness of life, celebrating life. Breathe in, drawing that energy into the centre of your chest, in the area of your heart. Feel your heart expand with your breath, and get hot, full of passion for life and love. Allow the fire to burn in your heart, burning away any obstacles to love.

- Pull the energy into the crown area at the top of your head. Imagine that you are growing branches, energetic branches reaching up into the sky. Feel these energetic channels reaching into the cool white fire of the universe – the realm beyond mortal life, the realm of the infinite, and of spirit.

- Draw the cool white fire of the infinite down through the branches into the crown at the top of your head. Open up your crown area to allow the cool white fire of the universe to rain down on your head like sparks. Feel the sense of infinite possibilities for you, the sense of spaciousness, of expansion.

- Bring this sense of spaciousness into your chest. Let your heart be soothed by this sense of spaciousness, allow your heart to open up. Imagine the cool white fire of the heavens burning together with the hot red fire of earth in your heart – mixing and mingling in the heat. See your heart as the centre of convergence, whose roots connect with the earth and whose branches connect with heaven. You are a bridge between the two. Celebrate these two qualities: your connection with the earth, your body and the material world, and your connection with the world of spirit.

- As you breathe out, allow the energy of this red and white heat to expand, allowing a sense of love to fill your heart. Allow this feeling of love to flow out from your heart towards your partner, and from your partner to the whole world beyond. As you breathe out, imagine love flowing out of you, as you breathe in, imagine receiving love. Breathe in and out, receiving and giving love.

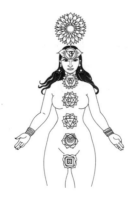

PURIFIYING THE CHAKRAS

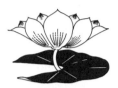

You can experience many different things in making love on different levels;
If I make love to a woman at a base level I feel myself affirmed because I've 'conquered' a woman.
If I make love at the level of the second chakra, I release my tension.
At the third level I experience my own energy and power which I keep in my own being.
At the fourth level I feel love.
At the level of the higher chakras, I experience a merging, with my partner, and through her to the universe.
By surrendering to my partner I become more than myself.

John Hawken

Purification is self-knowing. In becoming aware of how you are using your energy at all the different levels of the chakras, you can cleanse them. After reading through this list, jot down any issues that you're aware may be appropriate to you.

You can use your breath as a means of cleansing the chakras, using the model of the fire breath below, in which the fire burns away impurities and obstacles. Concentrate on letting go of the relevant issues when you are focusing on that particular chakra:

- At the level of the base chakra, purification involves letting go of issues around survival and insecurity, and understanding that we are all connected. If you're not aware of that you may be seeking security through sex.

- At the level of the second chakra, you can get hooked up on issues around power in relationships. Purification involves letting go of manipulation, and power over the other person. It means seeing relationships as an energy exchange, rather than an exchange involving money, goods or sex. Once you've done this, you can get to a position of honouring the other person for their essential self.

- The third chakra reflects issues around your relationship with yourself. If you are unable to say either no or yes clearly, because you don't know what you really want, you will need to do some self-discovery. Work on this chakra to clear the blocks to a healthy sense of self. The yin-yang game can be a helpful tool in learning how to honour yourself, as can self-pleasuring (page 175).

- The fourth chakra mediates between body and spirit. Purifying this chakra involves the ability to forgive, and learning how to behave with love and compassion.

- The fifth chakra is connected with creativity and expression, which is linked to the willpower. Here, the art of purification is about letting go of personal willpower, which is in the service of the self-centred ego, and aligning one's will with the divine. When you are truly aligned with the divine, there is no sense of separation between yourself and the divine, and you can act on your deepest desires from a place of congruence.

- The sixth chakra is connected with vision, and it is the centre that links the mind and the psyche. When you're stuck here you can be stuck in your head, rather than accessing true wisdom. In purifying this chakra you develop skill in evaluating beliefs and attitudes (rather than taking anything on faith), and developing what Buddhists would call an 'impersonal mind' which is objective and non-judgemental. This involves letting go of your own personal illusions and limited mind-set.

- The seventh chakra is traditionally thought of as the locus of your spiritual connection – the energy point for your life force. This is about the sense of meaning and purpose to your human existence, and purifying it involves developing devotional capacities.

ANOINTING THE CHAKRAS

This practice involves touching and visualizing the chakras in yourself and your partner using essential oils. Margo Anand, founder of SkyDancing training, suggested the oils below, but you can experiment with finding your own. You can use a single oil or mix them together in any combination you like.

Your partner lies down naked in a warm and comfortable nest. You need some small discs of absorbent paper on which you can place a drop or two each of the following essential oils:

Base:	ylang-ylang
Navel:	sage or cedar
Solar plexus:	tiger balm
Heart:	rose
Throat:	eucalyptus
Third eye:	mint
Crown:	lavender or rose.

Place a drop of the first essential oil on one of the seven paper circles. Kneeling beside your beloved, inhale the odour of the ylang-ylang oil for the base chakra, absorbing it and sending the smell sensation down into your own base chakra. Your partner can watch as you do this, 'seeing' the movement of energy into your base chakra. Next, reverentially waft the circle under their nose, allowing them to inhale and appreciate the sensation produced by this smell. As they inhale the odour down into the base chakra, lightly place the paper with the essential oil at the area of the base chakra (on the pubic hair – don't worry that you can't position it exactly).

Next, place a drop of the second essential oil on another paper circle. Inhale the sage aroma, drawing the smell sensation from your nose and lungs into your second chakra, while your beloved gazes into your eyes, sharing this process. Then place the circle in the region of the second chakra, in the area of the uterus, around 2–3 fingers below the belly button.

Continue in the same way until you have anointed all seven chakras.

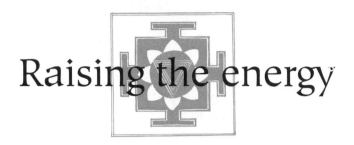

Raising the energy

To directly experience the energy Tantrics talk about can be easy. Just sit with your right hand held slightly away from your body. Shake it out vigorously, shaking out all the tension of the day. Let your hand shake loosely for at least 30 seconds. When you stop shaking, hold it out in front of you, next to your other hand. You'll notice that while your left hand feels inert and even dead, your right hand feels alive, warm, tingling, dynamic – in a word, energized. It's that easy to energize the body. So one good and simple way to energize your body is just to stand up with your feet a comfortable distance apart, bend your knees slightly, and just shake. Shake your whole body, getting rid of tension and tightness wherever you feel it in your body.

It can be very helpful to have some fast, dynamic music on that encourages you to shake out and shake loose. Shake your pelvis, letting your buttocks go wobbly. Shake your shoulders, letting your arms hang freely. Shake your head gently, easing out your neck and jaw. You may want to make a noise, freeing up your jaw and throat. Shake for up to ten minutes, before letting the wilder movements of your shaking gradually become smaller and smaller, leaving a fine shaking that feels like energy streaming through your body – just as you noticed after you finished shaking your right hand.

Now your body is loosened up, it can be good to dance. Just put on any music that you enjoy, and have a good bop. Tantrics prefer to energize the body in this way, before going on to meditation or visualization, ensuring that the body is charged up with energy rather than static. The feeling of vital energy this creates can be used in Tantric practices to expand your awareness.

FIRE MEDITATION

This meditation is good to cleanse your chakras. Fire has long been used by Tantrics as a symbol for burning away all impurities and obstructions on the spiritual path. Once you are familiar with the meditation, it is good to use some dynamic music to help you get into the dynamic mood of this meditation. Tantra teacher Leora Lightwoman suggests the first track on *Transfer Station Blue* by Michael Shrieve (see music resources). You can lead your partner through the meditation, or put it on tape for your own use.

- Stand with your spine straight and your feet planted on the floor, in alignment with your shoulders. Imagine you are sending roots down into the earth, through your feet.

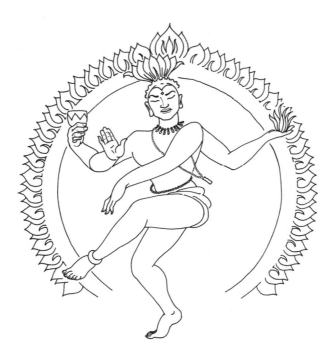

- Draw up the energy into your anus and genitals. The energy of the red fiery flame. Imagine this flame is licking up into your genitals burning away any sexual trauma or grief. Imagine this fiery red flame is consuming your legs and your pelvis. Imagine you are becoming the fire, the flame. Allow yourself to move and dance as that flame of pure energy.

- Then, as the flame climbs higher towards your navel, imagine the flame becoming bright orange. It consumes your pelvis and navel, burning away any creative blocks and cleansing your creative energy.

- Imagine this purifying flame climbing up to your solar plexus, clearing away the old in its voracious tongues of pure yellow flame.

- As more and more of your body is consumed imagine the flame becoming a brilliant green, as it licks the inside of your chest, burning away any grief and wounds in your heart, cleansing and opening your heart.

- This rainbow fire becomes blue as it burns away all the old blocks around your throat, clearing any problems with self-expression, and purifying this area of communication.

- The flames become violet as they consume your third eye area, burning out old redundant ways of viewing the world and others, and purifying and cleansing your vision. Imagine the flames as a rainbow of fiery flames licking up to the crown of your head, gradually becoming white.

- Allow yourself to dance as the flame, breathing, reaching from your passion into the realm of spirit. Feel yourself open to spirit.

- Then let the white flame subside, leaving you cleansed and purified. Let the white flame blend with the purple as it subsides into the area of the third eye, leaving a sense of space, vision and clarity.

- As it comes down through your throat imagine the flame turning blue, and leaving space for clearer communication.

- As the flame comes down into your heart, imagine it turning green, leaving a feeling of greater openness. In the solar plexus, where the yellow fire was, now there is your own brilliant sense of presence and empowerment.

- In the second chakra, imagine the flames becoming orange, leaving your sexuality cleansed and renewed.

- As the flame subsides into bright red tongues licking the base of your spine, it leaves you with an openness and connection to your life force, and a passion for life.

STREAMINGS

These exercises are a good preparation for opening your body to orgasmic response.

Elena, 50: Once I focused on letting go of my negative feelings they just washed through me and then something completely different was uncovered. The only way I can describe it is a holy magnet inside. I don't know why those words came back to me from an old Van Morrison song, but it felt like something pure and divine inside my vagina. All that 'victim' stuff had been covering up this golden magnet, stopping the magnet from doing it's work of attracting a partner – as well as other positive experiences in life.

The inside of my vagina felt so soft and silky. I've never ever experienced anything so soft. It's indescribable. That softness moved up from my vagina, through my inner flute. It was the exquisite softness of femininity. I'd always associated femininity with something weak, but this sensation was both powerful and incredibly soft. It made me realise how hard I'd become, dealing with pain and difficulties in life.

It was the most incredible state of ecstasy I've ever experienced. It was like an orgasm but somehow much more fine. It made every sexual experience I've ever had seem more gross.

I felt I was releasing this energy inside myself, accessing something deeper in me. Now I can tune into this feeling by focusing on my yoni – I get a sensation of fine energy streaming up through my chakras. If I'm lying in a warm bath with essential oils, and the water is touching my yoni, I can feel this aspect of my femininity coming back. I just need to trust it.

Kundalini shaking

This a simple way to raise energy in your body.

Close your eyes. Stand with spine upright and arms relaxed by your side. Stand with knees bent. Bending them stresses the thighs and calves, which produces tiny tremors after a few minutes of holding this position. To increase the sensation, you can rock very gently, with very small movements, forwards and backwards on the soles of your feet, changing the weight distribution on your feet ever so slightly. If you hold yourself at the edge of

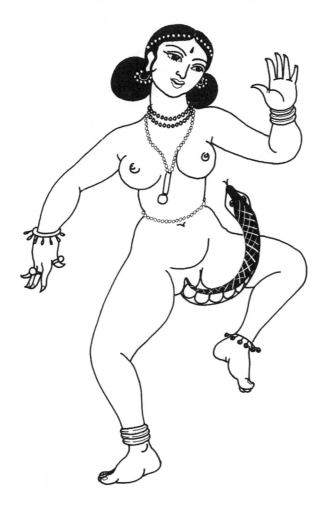

what feels comfortable for you, either forwards or backwards, you will experience more of these tremors.

Once these have started, you just hold that position and feel the sensations. As they build up, and before they become uncomfortable, let the trembling gradually expand up your legs and thighs, and into your genitals and pelvis. The tremblings may feel very fine and small, or they may feel strong and almost uncontrollable. However they feel, don't try and control them, just allow them to happen. Try not to change your position unless you feel very uncomfortable. If you can't hold the position move gently into a position of slightly less stress and try to hold that, rather than breaking the exercise by abruptly changing position completely.

If you want to, you can explore amplifying the movement, going with it. You breathe more deeply, or release whatever sound arises spontaneously. Keep the rest of your body relaxed, and especially your jaw. Feel the trembling spreading from your pelvis into your abdomen. If you can't feel this, shake your pelvis, loosely, or vigorously.

Pelvic bouncing

Get comfortable lying on your back, on a thick quilt on the floor.

Let the small of your back rest on the floor, and lengthen your neck, relaxing your jaw and shoulders. Your arms feel most comfortable lying by your sides, palms up. Lie with your knees bent, allowing your pelvis to move around freely. Make sure your shoulders are not crunched up, or your neck straining as you raise your pelvis off the floor.

Start with bouncing your pelvis up and down, breathing deeply as you do so. Experiment with different speeds and different degrees of vigorousness.

Just allow any vibrations that arise around your pelvis to move up your body.

Butterfly

The aim of this exercise is to focus on the energy streamings that arise around your pelvis and genitals. It is important to be able to allow energy to move in your pelvis, clearing any blocks to experiencing pleasure and the movement of energy during love-making.

Lie on your back. Bring your knees up bent, and then allow the knees to open out, to a point where they just feel comfortable.

Don't let them flop right outwards, just hold them open, allowing yourself to feel the small tremors in your thighs that are a sign of muscle tension. Instead of moving away from the tremors, stay with them and relax into them. Adjust your position to move in tiny movements around this area of slight strain and tension – exploring what the sensations feel like, and how to accentuate it.

This is a way of learning to relax into tension, rather than turn away from it, just as you do in orgasm. It's a way of allowing sensation and muscle release to happen in your body, without being in conflict. If you find this difficult, try saying 'yes' out loud each time you open out your legs, allowing the energy to arise. If you do this exercise with your partner present, it's good to have them sitting by your side, gazing into your eyes as you experience opening up and relaxing into the streaming of energy. Allowing your partner to witness this opening up is a privilege for them, and brings you into much greater intimacy.

Let the energy spread from your pelvis, thighs and sex up your body. Allow the sensation to spread out from your abdomen, and using your hand, and your breath, sweep or draw the energy up into your heart. If your partner is present, you can make a gesture of offering this energy to them, through your heart centre.

Gerhardt, 43: We were lying down together, moving and rocking our pelvises to energize the base chakra. At the same time I was drawing energy up from the base chakra with my breath and my hand, connecting my sexuality with my heart. Normally I feel a bit sick and dizzy, but I gave in to the movements, and I felt my pelvis lifting off the mattress with a feeling of ease.

The music had a strong effect on me, once my heart felt involved. It seemed to stir my heart and it helped open me up emotionally. With this soft music a sense of joy spread through my body, especially in my heart. The feeling was "Everything is perfect". It felt like I'd experienced a sliver of paradise. Everything was just the way I wanted it to be.

My partner was lying next to me with a beaming open smile, and smiling eyes. We fell into each other's arms with such complete ease – all the barriers just dropped away and we connected on a deep level in complete harmony. Whatever we did, we moved together in a feeling of high energy.

Often as a man I feel the impulses coming from me, I end up leading. I like more sense of equality, and for women to initiate. I like to be either passive or active equally, according to the situation. But this time we went beyond all that. There didn't seem to be anyone leading, or sometimes I felt she was subtly leading me. We looked into each other's eyes – it felt like a direct contact with another soul, going beyond personality.

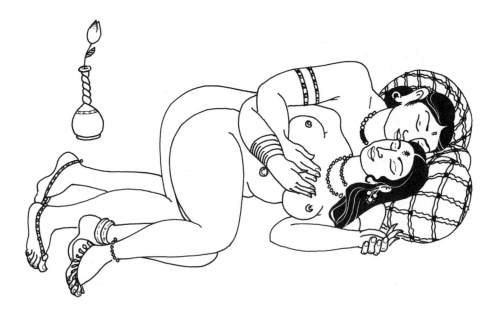

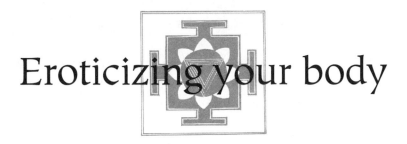

Eroticizing your body

Martin 45: There's a sense of all my body being present and alive, not just the bit I can feel at the moment. It's not buzzy, just tingly, as if I'm more aware than usual. I feel it all over, in my toes, in my elbows. It's all over, not just in my genitals.

These exercises heighten sensitivity and awareness, and help to open the body and mind to love and excitement. Moving from the drive for sensation, into opening to sensitivity. You need to prepare for the exercise beforehand so that your partner can just relax and concentrate on what is happening in the present moment, without thoughts or expectations. These exercises are designed to be done by one of you first, before swapping roles.

AWAKENING THE SENSES

In this exercise each partner introduces the other to a range of sensory experiences beyond the scope of ordinary sensory perceptions. Each of the five senses is stimulated in turn. Awaken the sense of hearing (music), smell (scents and essential oils), taste (fruit), touch (stroking with feathers) and sight (remove the blindfold to look at each other, and the beautiful objects your partner has arranged). Your partner should be blindfolded so there are no distractions, and it's also best not done on a full stomach.

Light candles and incense and put the food tray in the centre of the room, along with all the other objects you will use. You can create a pleasing arrangement of all the objects you will use, as well as flowers and other beautiful things that have meaning for you both. Blindfold your partner and gently lead him into the room, saying that there is no need to talk. Explain he doesn't need to do anything but breathe deeply, relax and enjoy the experiences you offer them. Spend about an hour on this exercise, leaving a minute or so between each stimulus.

- Hearing: If you have any musical instruments such as bells, cymbals, flutes or maracas you can use these. Begin by introducing just one sound – as continuous and resonant as possible. For instance, ring a bell, moving it around your partner while it is still ringing. You can use unusual sounds, like scraping or scrunching – preferably sounds that are not immediately recognisable so that your partner isn't distracted from listening to the sound by working out what's producing it. Otherwise use short excerpts of beautiful and interesting music. Choose your favourite atmospheric music; it should be gentle and relaxing or lyrical.

- Smell: Pass perfumes and essential oils under your partner's nose without touching the skin. Allow them to inhale, and then a wait a minute or more before offering the next smell, particularly if the odour is lingering. Peppermint or eucalyptus essence is good to start with, after that, use sweeter and more mysterious essences such as ylang-ylang and gardenia. Play music that incorporates the sound of running water or splashes of waves, and spray a fine mist of scented water like rosewater over their head.

- Taste: Playfully offer small mouthful-sized portions of exotic fruit, like avocado, mango, star fruit, passion or kiwifruit to your partner's mouth. Rub their lips with the morsel, teasing and tantalising their taste-buds. Offer a glass of sparkling elderflower wine or cordial (you'll need a straw for your partner to take a sip while still blind-folded), or drip a drop of honey on their lips. After a minute offer the next taste sensation. For example, you can dip a grape into liqueur and let your partner smell it. After a moment caress the lips with the grape before teasingly offering it to their mouth – and finally press it to the lips until they part and allow it to go in ever so slowly. You can dip your finger into the liqueur and caress your partner's lips with it.

- Touch: Brush the skin first with a piece of fur, then with feather, silk or other textured fabrics. Move the fabric extremely slowly and deli-cately across the cheeks, neck and arms – or wrists and ankles. You can use your hair to tickle their skin, or blow gently in unexpected places. If you use your fingertips or nails, keep your touch very light and fine – and your movements very slow, because that enhances the sensitivity of your partner's experience of touch.

- After a moment's silence change the music to something that makes you both feel full of love. Sitting behind your partner, gently rest your hand on his heart. Allow them to lean back on you, feeling your warmth.

- Sight: To close the ritual, silently remove your partner's blindfold and look at each other, and the objects you have used. Close the ritual with a long, tender hug.

DANCE OF THE GODDESS

Chakra Sambhara Tantra

Visualize yourself as an erotic red goddess; symbol of dedication and passion. Three eyes blazing with passion; your tongue is lustful, with the purifying power of your inner fire. As goddess you are naked, with dishevelled hair; symbolizing freedom from the bonds of delusion. You are intuition – a reminder that every-thing must pass. Blazing like a fire you express your wisdom essence, in embrac-ing your lover without restraint.

Invoking Kundalini – your inner woman

This exercise follows the previous one perfectly. Here you are invited to explore your own beauty and self-worth; expressing yourself through dance. Discuss who should go first. It may be easier for whoever enjoys dancing more to start. Remember that there are no rules on how a goddess or god would or should dance. Just as there are many different aspects of deity, repre-sented by different goddesses and gods, there are many different moods that can be expressed in the dance. Just enjoy exploring these different aspects, and don't worry about pleasing your part-ner. There is no right way to dance, but treat it as both seductive and playful, and reverential – as if you and your lover are Shakti and Shiva. Allow whatever moods come over you to emerge. Let yourself express your moods in your dancing. be provocative, be flirtatious, be serene, be wild ... be yourself.

You can start the dance with a salutation of greeting – bowing to your partner.

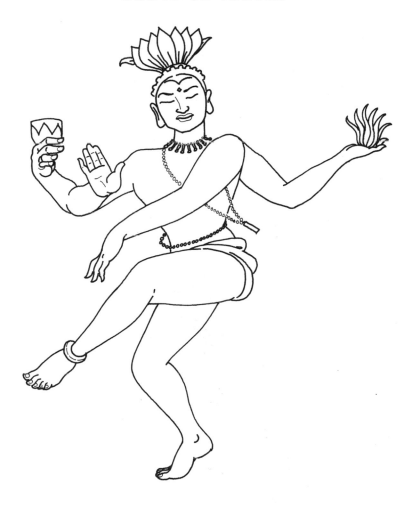

Your partner sits attentively in front of a stage area, and you enter wearing something comfortable that makes you feel beautiful – or perhaps just a skimpy scarf. Many men like to allow their lingam to dance freely, moving against their thighs. Dance naked if you want.

Using your favourite music, find your own unique style to dance for your partner. Choose pieces that last 15–20 minutes in total.

Hilary, Tantra teacher: One of the most powerful images that came to me was during a meditation on my introductory Taste of Tantra weekend. In my mind's eye I saw a woman dancing in front of other women. As she danced, she was taking off her clothes one by one, in the most beautiful way. I was struck by her grace, and by how much she was enjoying herself, and seemed to be totally in her body. I felt I would like to be that free, that I could immerse myself in the pleasure of that action. Then suddenly the woman came up close to me, and I saw that she was me! It was an image of what I would actually become.

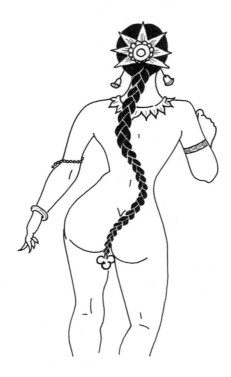

EROTIC TOUCH

Rediscover the art of sensual touch with your partner. You'll need some long delicate feathers, such as peacock feathers, as well as light scarves of different textures – say silk or velvet.

Play soft, sensual music. Your partner lies down naked in a warm room. Stroke your partner's body gently with a feather, starting around the shoulders and throat, then moving gradually and sensuously down the body to the feet, and finishing with the head. Then use your fingertips, and lastly your breath, blowing about an inch away from the body. Touch feels more lovely the slower and more continuous it is. Take your time, enjoying both giving and receiving without any goal.

You can also experiment with different textures – such as a soft, light silk or velvet drape to slowly and delicately touch your partner's skin. Hair also feels nice, slowly trailed across bare skin.

Keep your touch very light and as slow as possible. Treat your partner's body as a whole rather than focusing on erogenous zones. This is not a prelude to lovemaking, but fulfils the desire for sensual touch independent of sexual contact. For the giver, the mood is one of meditation rather than trying to excite or arouse your partner. Treat every part of your partner's bare skin with equal care and attention. The role of the receiver is just to relax and focus on the experience of receiving – without expectations about how it will feel. Use slow, calm breathing to stay in relaxation, and let go of any expectations or sense of having a goal. You should spend 20–40 minutes before swapping roles.

Whatever you do, do it consciously – that means with your full attention on what you are doing. Here are some different types of touch that you may like to try:

- scratching
- pressing
- circling
- jumping
- tracing a line
- pressing
- rubbing
- kissing

Be inventive with your mouth. Kissing and biting can be very pleasurable, for example lipping, tonguing, sucking, blowing. Discover different techniques for different parts of the body, for example, biting the nape of the neck, nibbling the pubic mound, caressing the breasts with a wide open mouth. Play with the base of spine, shoulders, left cheek, toes, breasts.

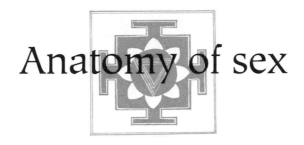

Anatomy of sex

THE LOVE MUSCLE

To explore the Tantric poles of expansion and contraction, experiment with contracting and releasing your PC muscles. Your PC
muscles form the floor of your pelvis, and they're the ones you
use to stop and start the flow of your pee. The anatomical name is
the pubococcygeal muscles, which many women are familiar with
because they usually need toning up after childbirth. In Tantra
they're called the love muscle, or fire muscle, because they can be
used to build up sexual energy in the body, or to relax into sexual
pleasure.

In breathing exercises, the love muscle can be squeezed on the
in-breath as you imagine energy being drawn up through the
energy channels of your body, helping to build up an energy
charge. If you can't feel your love muscle very easily, or it seems
weak, you'll need to practise doing at least 100 squeezes a day.
These are the same muscles that stop and start your flow of urine.
You can practise squeezing and strengthening them anywhere.

In this exercise you sit comfortably, upright, breathing in a
relaxed, even way. Breathe in, allowing the air to fill your lower
abdomen. Relax as you breathe out. Allow a sense of space in
your pelvis. Now, as you breathe in, squeeze your love muscles.
As you breathe out, relax the love muscles. Keep breathing in and
out, squeezing and relaxing your muscles.

Now, breathe out relaxing your love muscles, and breathe
in without contracting them. On the next out-breath, relax the

muscles even more. You'll notice that even when you think you're relaxed there's often the possibility of relaxing even more. Just notice if there is any holding on or tension, and breathe in and out again, allowing these muscles to deeply relax. When you're ready to finish, allow your awareness to spread through your whole body.

You can play with this short exercise, feeling the difference between doing, and not doing. Feeling how much letting go there is in relaxing.

FIRE MEDITATION WITH LOVE MUSCLE SQUEEZE

The aim of this meditation is to build onto the fire meditation you have already done, and include the love muscle squeeze. You visualize the flame in each chakra, for several breaths, co-ordinating the love muscle squeeze with each breath. The love muscle squeeze is thought by Tantrics to seal energy in your body, allowing the energy charge you are building to intensify.

- Lie on the floor with your knees raised. Lift your pelvis and start rocking and shaking it to build an energy charge in your sacrum.

- Keep breathing slowly and evenly as you feel the energy charge building up in your pelvis.

- With your back on the floor, introduce the love muscle (PC muscle) squeeze in time to your breath. Squeeze as you breathe in, release as you breathe out.

- Imagine a fiery red flame igniting at the base of your spine, around your perineum. Draw the red fiery energy of the flame into your base chakra, and allow it to subside on each exhalation. Squeeze the love muscle with each inhalation. After several breaths, you will draw the flame into the second chakra. You will then draw it from the base chakra into each successive chakra, allowing it to return to your base chakra on every exhalation.

  - After a few breaths imagine the red flame turning orange as you draw it up into the second chakra, in the navel, stoking the fire of your sexuality. On the next in-breath draw this flame up to your second chakra. Visualize the raw red flame spreading from your spine into your pelvis. Use your hand to stroke the flame along your skin from your genitals up to your navel. As you draw the flame up with your breath and hand, and clenched love muscle, imagine the orange flame feeding your creativity. As you stroke upwards, breathe in and squeeze the love muscle. As you breathe out release the squeeze and, with your hand, follow the energy returning back to the base chakra.

- As you exhale release the love muscle and trace the withdrawing orange flame back down to your base chakra with your hand.

- Next, as you draw the flame up to the third chakra, imagine the flames turning a vibrant yellow. Breathe these yellow flames into your navel, expanding out into your solar plexus, nourishing your sense of empowerment.

- Next, imagine the green flame entering your heart. Encourage the flame to climb, squeezing your love muscle as you inhale, gradually relaxing it as you exhale. Bring your hand up to your chest and hold the green flame in your heart, as you continue to pump energy into the heart region with your love muscle.

- Then imagine blue flames climbing up to your throat chakra. Help them climb with your hand, and your love muscle. Allow the flames to nurture this centre, nurturing your ability to express yourself on every level, and strengthening your powers to communicate clearly and effectively.

- The flames become violet as they consume your third eye chakra, purifying your vision. Continue working with the love muscle.

- Imagine the flames becoming white as they lick around the crown of your head.

- Then bring the healing white light down through each chakra, returning to the base of your spine.

Improving your sexual enjoyment

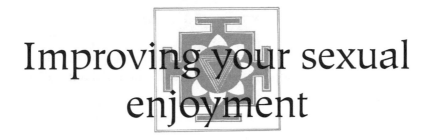

SELF PLEASURING

Pooja, 45: Doing Tantra I learnt different ways of pleasuring myself. To know that self-pleasure is okay. In some Asian families it's difficult for women to accept their sexual pleasure. Asian women are expected to look like goddesses, but they can't be sexual beings. Just to touch can be taboo. Many women can't enjoy even having their arm stroked. Sex is purely for procreation.

I've always felt desirable, but from 18 onwards I would not let a man near me, sexually. When my periods stopped early I felt this wasn't right, I'd lost my femininity.

Tantra is allowing me to become alive again, and accept sexual pleasure. In my dreams my body changes shape, and size. In my dreams I feel a sense of my body really relaxing. I have had dreams of a lovely warm vagina. I feel more positive. I'm aware of judgements, and how they stop me having pleasure.

Masturbation is not looked down on in Tantric sexual practices. Instead, it's considered essential for self discovery, learning about your own unique sexual response, and focusing in on the subtle sexual and sensual feelings you experience.

To learn Tantric techniques you need to become more aware of your own sexual response.

The best way to do that is to observe your own path to orgasm. It's easier to do this while masturbating, without the distraction of your partner around.

Self pleasuring is the foundation of sexual exploration and discovery. It enables you to get in touch with your own sexual needs, and encourages you to take responsibility for ensuring that these are met when you're making love with your partner. If you feel uncomfortable or ashamed about self-pleasuring, it's important to take time regularly to work on feeling comfortable about doing so, stripping off the layers of shame and guilt so many of us have built up around our sexual selves.

It is difficult to feel fully relaxed and open with another, so long as we still feel inhibited about our own pleasure – and it's also difficult for us to reach our full potential for pleasure if part of us is judging ourselves. As self-love, it's also a sign of making a commitment to yourself.

It can be utilized as a means of developing control over habitual sexual response. Self-pleasuring is a means to learn how to extend sexual pleasure and erotic sensations, and to develop an awareness of how sexual energy involves the subtle energies of the body. You can use self-pleasuring to draw together some of the practices you've been reading about in this book. You can practise breathing techniques, and sensing or visualizing the movement of energies through the inner flute.

Terry, 37: The self pleasuring started with dancing with myself, which felt wonderful, and then stripping off for myself. I felt completely free of any worries or inhibitions about myself, because I was wearing a blindfold. In my mind's eye, while the dancing was happening I saw my own face. I felt I was touching my face and holding my body as if I was my own lover. I saw an image of a green lake, and myself rising up out of the lake, looking beautiful and sexy and god-like. I connected with a part of me that was perfect and god-like. I felt whole and powerful and innocent, all at the same time. I felt completely sexy and gorgeous.

Self pleasuring was very powerful: the biggest experience of loving myself physically, and spending a long time exploring my own body as a lover would. I got lost in myself almost like a meditation, it was so peaceful and relaxing.

I also discovered some new feelings in my genitals. I stroked myself from the perineum forwards and up over my testicles, which I'd never done before. It felt beautiful. I explored the head of my penis with lubricant. Before I'd found it too much, too intense, almost unbearable

The feeling started to space me out and go up through my heart and out through my head like an intense beam of energy. I achieved a deep connection with myself during dance, much less shame during striptease, and no shame at all about self-pleasuring. I played with myself for two hours and didn't feel the slightest need to ejaculate. I was completely enjoying the feelings, the thought of ejaculating didn't seem to be there.

I enjoyed playing without having a full erection, exploring new feelings. I'd never taken the time to do it. The areas around the inside of my thighs and buttocks and perineum felt exquisitely sensual rather than sexual. It was the most amazing experience of loving myself. I felt calm and relaxed and happy and powerful at the same time. I looked like a warrior afterwards.

HONOURING YONI

The aim of this exercise is to really look at and appreciate Shakti's yoni, honouring her genitals as divine. For the receiver, it is a very profound experience of being seen:

- Bring a gift or offering to present to the yoni; it could be a flower or a shell that reminds you of the yoni, or it could be something that you know yoni likes. It is important to maintain frequent eye contact. Your partner needs to see the love in your eyes. Look at yoni with reverence and wonder. Many women are ashamed or embarrassed about their genitals, and feel discomfort when they are looked at. It's important to take the time to look. Even where couples often have oral sex, they may not be used to their genitals just being looked at and appreciated.

- For the woman, it's also an important exercise for deepening trust. It's important to feel you are in charge of your boundaries, and to tell your partner if there's anything you don't like him doing. It's important to keep your channels of communication open, and not feel as if anything is being done to you that you don't want. If you are happy with the way your lover is honouring your yoni, you can just relax into receiving his loving attention.

- With your partner sitting with her legs wide open, leaning back on some comfortable cushions and gazing at you, kneel before yoni, and bow before yoni, presenting your gift.

- Gaze at yoni, taking time to really look, and then tell your partner what you see, and what you like about what you see. Really take in how yoni looks, and look in your partner's eyes when you tell her.

- For some people this will be enough, especially the first time you do this exercise.

- But if your partner feels it's appropriate, she may invite you to touch her yoni. Your touch should be extremely gentle and reverential. You're not aiming to excite her, but to explore her. To really feel the different parts of her yoni: the pubic hair, the inner and outer lips, her pearl (clitoris), vaginal entrance, perineum (towards the anus) and rosetta (anus) if your partner likes. Ask her if what you're doing is okay.

- You can kiss yoni with kisses and licks. The receiver can experience just relaxing and receiving these different touches, without feeling she must get aroused – and without feeling she mustn't.

- Again experience what this feels like, and really taste yoni. It is part of Tantric practices to absorb the sexual fluids of women, as well as the fluids emanating from their breasts, and the menstrual blood.

- You may want to extend this exercise by honouring yoni with your lingam, by laying it against yoni (externally).

- If, and only if, your partner invites you in, just stay still inside her without moving much, because that feels more like a healing presence.

Rachel 37: During the yoni talk – where we gave our genitals a voice – I was surprised at what came out. I cried a lot with deep sobs. I've had hormonal problems all my life, which I eventually got sorted with homeopathy, and I realized how painful that had been.

Through moving my body a lot I found I could let go of restrictions. When something painful came up I noticed I wasn't breathing properly. So I learnt to breathe into that, and I could feel I was letting go of another layer of constrictions.

HONOURING LINGAM

Sally, 29: There's a subtle distinction between doing something because I should, and doing something because it really is sacred. It's not about martyrdom, it really is about seeing the sacred in another.

If I'm pleasuring my partner's lingam, I like to do it because I feel loving and honouring of him, rather than because I want to give him a good time. So in honouring, it's important that whatever I'm doing, I'm doing it from my heart. And as he's experiencing pleasure in his sex, I'm experiencing pleasure in my heart. Of course, that energy spreads and permeates through the body. His sexual pleasure spreads up to his heart, and my heart pleasure spreads to my sex.

The aim of this exercise is to honour Shiva's lingam in its natural state. This allows him to experience his lingam in a different way from normal – not as an instrument he should be ready to use,

nor as something he feels ambivalent or ashamed of. The honouring allows him to be visible, and for his genitals to be really seen.
Your intention is very important here, and it's important not to
step over the boundaries of the exercise so that the man can really
let go and relax into the experience.

Another aim of this exercise is to break down the association
of erection with arousal and readiness for intercourse. Whether
erection is there or not, honour your partner's lingam without
trying to excite it. It is lovely for a man to have his
penis touched while soft: a completely different
experience, which may put him in touch with qualities of vulnerability or innocence. Keep eye contact, because this is about connecting and
honouring, not stimulating your partner.

Just as Tantrics honour the yoni-lingam, washing, anointing and garlanding the lingam with
flowers, so you can honour your partner's
lingam. With your partner sitting with his legs
wide open, leaning back on some comfortable
cushions and gazing at you, kneel before lingam,
and bow before lingam, presenting your gift.

Gaze at lingam, taking time to really look, and then tell
your partner what you see, and what you like about what you
see. Really take in how his lingam looks, and look in your partner's eyes when you tell him.

If your partner feels it's appropriate, he may invite you to
touch his lingam. Your touch should be extremely gentle and reverential. You're not aiming to excite him, but to explore him.
Explore his pubic area, his scrotum, and perineum, and his
lingam. Check that your touch is okay. Explore different touches.
Use a light touch, especially around the scrotum, and hold his
balls delicately, as if they were eggs. Stroke and massage the

sensitive skin of the testicles, blow on the delicate skin around the testicles and perineum – then try taking his scrotum into your mouth.

Finger the shaft of your partner's lingam as if it were a flute. Travel around the lingam, avoiding the usual up and down stroking that mimics intercourse. The aim is not to excite and bring your partner to orgasm, but to honour and respect his lingam.

HEALING YONI MASSAGE

Michaela, 43: I was attracted to Tantra because I was looking for sexual healing. I couldn't allow anything to penetrate me, and for years I had a relationship with a woman. But it bothered me that I seemed to have so much fear in my yoni. I saw a psychosexual therapist, and she was trying to accustom me to allow my vaginal muscles to relax, gradually bringing a finger closer and closer, telling me that it was my choice, and that at any stage I could stop.

On the Tantra training we did a yoni healing, where my yoni was massaged by one person in a healing, non-sexual way, while another two people were there to support me. Just the thought of something entering me would bring up so much fear, and I was absolutely terrified at what would happen to me. I kept saying, 'help me, help me' to my partner, and I had to look into her eyes to find an anchor. I really thought I wouldn't survive the experience.

What came up was unexpected. I had vague memories of oral abuse with my brother, whom I loved dearly. When I was 21 I lost him suddenly – he died in front of me of a heart attack when we were playing tennis. I broke off with my boyfriend soon after because I couldn't have sex with him. I realized that I was holding onto a lot of shock in my vagina.

When my brother died, I had wanted to scream but couldn't, and what happened after that yoni healing, next day, was that I screamed for several minutes. Since then I find I can cry more freely, and I'm not so afraid. In a way, Tantra has opened up old wounds – which feels okay, because they were slowly eating away at me. Now, with more support, I can choose to heal them.

The purpose of the yoni massage is to heal the memories of past experiences stored in the yoni. Because old experiences can be stored in the tissues as cellular memories, make sure to create a sacred space before this exercise, and to really connect with your partner. Make sure that every movement and every touch is gentle and loving. Encourage her to breathe into the experience by deepening your own breathing. If your partner does get upset, ask her what she needs from you. Ask her if she wants you to carry on, stay exactly as you are, or to stop and just hold her.

Communication is very important in this massage; Shakti needs to let you know what she likes and doesn't like, and to share with you any feelings that come up for her. If she doesn't want to talk too much during the massage, she can share afterwards:

- Your partner should lie comfortably on her back, with pillows under her head and anywhere else she needs them. You can sit by her side, or between her open legs, which are also supported by cushions. Gaze at your partner and harmonize your breath with hers, establishing a loving heart connection. Gently rest your left hand on her heart centre, while your right hand (if you are right-handed) rests on her pelvis, over her sacral chakra.

- After a few minutes, start to massage her whole body, with oil or talc if you want to use it. You can brush energy away from the pelvis area, upwards toward the abdomen and down the arms as well as down her thighs and legs.

- Massage around her pelvis, the band of muscles along the top of her pubic area, and along her groin (the crease where her thighs meet her pubic area), and the tops of her thighs – all areas where tension can be held. Check the pace and pressure of your massage movements with her.

- Just before you start the yoni massage, cup your hand over the pubic area and lips of the yoni, again holding your hand over her heart centre and re-establishing eye connection.

- After gently stroking the pubic area, pour a small quantity of a good lubricant around the outer lips of the yoni, and begin gently massaging the fleshy parts. Spend some time here and do not rush. Look at your partner's yoni, and admire it, and say what you see.

- Gently squeeze the outer lip between your thumb and forefinger, and slide up and down the entire length of each lip. Do the same thing to the inner lips of the yoni (vulva). Then gently squeeze all the lips together between your hands, in a yoni sandwich. Check with your partner that she is enjoying the pace and pressure of your touch.

- Gently stroke the clitoris with small circles and gentle squeezes. Encourage your partner just to relax into any erotic sensations, without focusing too much on them. You can disperse energy by stroking it away from the pelvis again, or you can build energy with blended stimulation – stroking and circling a nipple with your free hand.

- When your partner is ready, she will invite you to slowly slide the middle finger of your right hand inside her vagina. Begin to gently explore the inside of the vagina in every direction, and massage it. The rest of your hand can rest on or massage the pubic mound. Vary the depth, speed and pressure of your fingers. There are three main types of movement: small circles, vibrating on any areas that feel numb, and just holding, particularly if your partner gets distressed (it's better to stay still, without withdrawing).

- With your palm facing up, and the middle finger inside the yoni, move the middle finger in a 'come here' gesture or crook back towards the palm. You will contact a spongy area of tissue just under the pubic bone, behind the clitoris. This is the G-spot, or in Tantra, the sacred spot. Your partner may feel as if she has to urinate or it may be painful or pleasurable. Stop moving your finger if it feels uncomfortable to your partner or try varying the pressure, speed and pattern of movement. You can move side to side, back and forth, or in circles with your middle finger.

- Keep breathing and looking into each other's eyes. Powerful emotions may come up and she may well cry, or want to share what's coming up. Just keep breathing and be gentle. Don't panic. Keep massaging until she tells you to stop. Very slowly, gently, and with respect, remove your hands. Allow her to just lay there and enjoy the afterglow of the yoni massage. Cuddling or holding is very soothing as well.

MASSAGING THE LINGAM

Paul, 52: I don't like my lingam being pounced on with the aim of being pleasured. What I like is a gradual process of allowing myself to relax into a state of receptivity.

I prefer to be lightly and gently stroked all over my body until my skin becomes more and more sensitive. Lightly stroking my nipples and my genitals as well but not focusing on these areas.

The more slowly and delicately my partner touches me, the more relaxed I feel and the more pleasure I feel. My skin becomes more sensitive and I gradually plateau in a feeling of relaxation. I have a sense of stillness in my body, and the more still my body becomes the more powerful the sensations are. When I feel I've reached this place of total surrender – that's when I like my lingam to be pleasured.

I like my whole penis to be stroked, including my balls. Usually my penis is soft and I lie quite still, though sometimes I like to roll my pelvis around and arch my back or squeeze something in my hands.

I like the whole head of my penis to be pleasured, and there's a particular place just under the tip of my penis where the foreskin joins it that I love to be touched. It seems to switch on a light in my forehead and I lose awareness of my penis. All my attention focuses on the middle of my forehead, filling my consciousness. I have a sense of openness in my head, a feeling of more space inside and on either side of my head, expansion. It's a really deep stillness. I suppose it's ecstasy. I don't know where I am and it's timeless.

Now I can pleasure myself with this slow gentle touch, and a soft penis – it feels more pleasurable than friction.

But if my partner is touching me, it's really important for me to have eye contact with my partner, to feel connected with her, which helps me to melt into her.

Old patterns don't just drop away immediately. It's taken me three years to get to this state. It would take me an hour or so of being touched and stroked just to relax, and I used to ask my partner to rub my penis till I got to the point of orgasm and then stop, and I'd do this a few times until I broke through the need to have an orgasm and learnt to let go of it. It was a revelation to me to learn that I could be pleasured in any other way but the way I'd known for the last 30 years.

When my penis is pleasured without me being in this state of relaxation it remains a purely physical pleasure and it's confined to my penis. It feels nice, and it's erotic, but it makes me want to do more and more, I want more friction and harder, and I feel I need to do something to increase the pleasure, tensing my body and building up a lot of pressure that needs to be released.

The aim of this massage is to experience letting go and relaxing into sensations. Just allow yourself to feel your responses, without feeling you have to do anything about them. It's very important to learn to receive. There is too much emphasis in male sexuality on having to perform, and viewing the penis as performer. Your lingam does not have to be ready to perform at any time. It's sometimes a relief to experience your lingam as just being – not being anything in particular. You can also allow yourself to experience the different feelings and moods of your lingam, and it doesn't matter whether you have an erection, or you don't have an erection, at any stage of this massage. Your lingam can be shy, ardent, playful, proud, fiery or full of shame. Again, you may find that having your lingam touched in a gentle, non-threatening way, releases cellular memories, and you may want to hold the massage right there, or stop it and just be held by your partner. If so, your massage should follow the pattern of the healing yoni massage rather than the lingam massage that follows.

Another aspect of this lingam massage is allowing your erotic energy to spread out from your genitals. In order to prepare for the experience of whole body orgasm, as opposed to a genital orgasm, you need to learn to feel the sensations throughout your body, not just your lingam, and to connect your sexual energy with your heart, and with your spirituality. One of the best ways to do this is to give up your attachment to orgasm, in order to allow yourself to experience extended pleasure. The lingam massage is also about celebrating your lingam as a source of pleasure, and allowing yourself to experience that pleasure.

Exercise

- Cuddle, and create a heart connection, placing your hand over your partner's heart chakra, and sending your energy into his heart, through your breath.

- Allow your partner to melt into you, relaxing and opening himself up to receive. If this makes him feel vulnerable, allow that. Mother his inner child, if that's what he wants.

- To energise his pelvis, Shiva lifts his buttocks off the floor and shakes them. You can help release the muscles by jiggling his buttocks, or giving the muscles light, energizing massage strokes to free them up.

- As he shakes, encourage the energy to ground itself by stroking it down his thighs and legs, into his feet. You can put your hands over his feet.

- Then as he settles, place one hand on his sacrum, above the chakra, and one over his heart chakra, connecting them together in his awareness. Align your breathing with his, slowing down and taking time. This stage is about relaxing into the sensations he has created by releasing tension and stimulating energy.

- Massage the muscles which support the pelvic floor. Start with the muscles at the base of the abdomen – just above his pubic hair – then massage down into his groin. (Be careful of lymph glands here, which can sometimes feel a bit tender – if so don't massage them.) Work in a U shape, from the crest of one hip into the crest of the other. Massage down into his thighs – you can usually press quite deeply here.

- Massage behind his testicles, in and around them. Ask your partner what kind of pressure he likes – usually this area can take a firm touch. Massage around the perineum, and deep into the tissue as far as you can. This is the area where the spongy tissues of the base of the penis go deep into the pelvic floor.

- Cradle a testicle in one hand. Hold it very delicately for some minutes – many men are uncomfortable at first at having their testicles handled. Shiva, you can relax into a sense of trust, as your partner gently takes the weight of your balls, one at a time.

- You can take the skin of the scrotum in your hand. Pull it away from the testicles and gently rub between your thumb and forefingers. Ask your partner what feels nice.

- Inside the scrotum you can feel the tube that carries the seminal fluid from the testicles to the penis, and it can be lightly stroked.

- Roots of the lingam. Where you feel a hollow in the bones of the sacrum, curl your fingers over the bone to work on the attachment of the muscles to the bone. Usually there's a lot of tension here, which can gently be released in this massage.

- Allow any erotic energy to arise, but don't encourage it or have it as an intent. Shiva, just breath into the energy, allowing yourself to experience any erotic sensations and feelings without feeling you have to do anything about them, or take charge of the situation. Stay with the experience of just receiving.

- If your partner gets aroused, help him to focus on dispersing the sexual energy away from his genitals by stroking the energy up his chest to his heart area. You can hold your hand over his heart chakra, gazing at him lovingly.

- Spread the energy across the chest right down to his fingertips, and down his thighs into his legs.

- Massage his lingam from the scrotum up. It is easier to massage when his lingam is soft or semi-erect rather than erect, because you can play with the loose skin more easily. If he is very aroused, move away from his lingam again, dispersing his genital excitement.

- Penis reflexology suggests that there are seven chakra points up the lingam. The area at the perineum corresponds to the base chakra. The second chakra is at the base of the penis, where it joins the scrotum. The area where foreskin joins glans (forming a v shape) corresponds to the brow chakra. The area at the top of the glans, where the pee exits, corresponds to the crown chakra. You can play with these chakra points by spreading your fingers in a ring around his penis, and gently squeezing and massaging your way up his lingam from the base. Don't worry too much about where the points are supposed to be, just massage at close intervals from the bottom to the top – he will tell you what feels good.

- Play with stimulating his lingam and sacred spot (deep in the perineum) at the same time. This is called blended stimulation, stimulating two erogenous zones at the same time.

- The goal of lingam massage is not orgasm – although it may happen. For both of you, it's important to try not to get attached to ejaculating or not. It is also helpful for the giver to not expect anything in return. Just allow the receiver to enjoy the massage and to relax into himself afterwards.

- If orgasm does occur it is usually more intense and more satisfying, and the sensations are expanded throughout the body.

Extended sexual pleasure

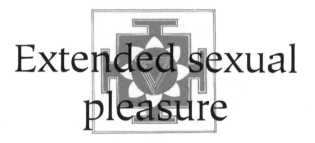

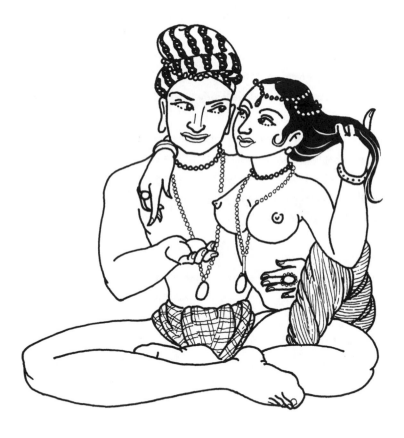

Karen, 43: Because my partner was able to make love for a long time without coming, we were able to reach extraordinary states of arousal. We had bursts of vigorous screwing, feeling very excited, but beyond the point of wanting to have an orgasm. My whole body felt alive and tingling, spreading out from my belly. We'd stop and lie together, with him still inside me, looking at each other. I felt a deep sense of peace, and of love. It was very joyful, and blissful, whether we were screwing, or lying exhausted together. Neither of us wanted to break it. I was having little orgasms throughout our love-making, and eventually after hours, he'd have an orgasm, and we would get some rest, feeling fully satisfied in a way I'd never felt before.

I felt as if I'd really been met for the first time, that we'd really connected in this prolonged state of arousal without end.

Now I feel I'm more sensitive, and I can't take that sort of intense friction of vigorous sex anymore. I understand more about the softness of opening out to him, and of slowness and sensuality. I feel deeply relaxed in my body now, and in touch with my own sensitivity.

Women's sexual experience is often divided into five levels of orgasmic experience. From pre-orgasmic, sporadically orgasmic, orgasmic and multiply orgasmic. The fifth level is called *extended sexual pleasure*, in which the orgasmic response is lengthened in order to prolong sexual pleasure. The following exercise aims to teach techniques for doing this, which can prepare you for the sixth stage, which Tantric practitioners call 'the wave of bliss'. The wave of bliss involves expanding extended sexual pleasure into an altered state of consciousness, using the breathing and visualization techniques we've been exploring throughout the book.

Tantric writings describe Shakti as achieving seven peaks of ecstasy, each peak higher, stronger, and more powerful than the preceding, until at the topmost she releases her nectar or amrita (female ejaculation).

Men's sexual experience is usually divided into the stages of arousal, build up to orgasm, orgasm and ejaculation.

Among advanced Tantric practitioners, these stages are separated. During extended sexual pleasuring men learn to peak and plateau again without going into orgasm. They then learn to orgasm without ejaculation, moving the subtle energies of sexual arousal away from the genitals and up through the inner flute. By moving energy away from the genitals, ejaculation may even disappear, but the body is capable of experiencing a whole body orgasm, in which erotic pleasure and the waves of energy produced in orgasm are diffused throughout the body.

Once you've gained the ability to orgasm without ejaculation, you can choose whether and when you'd like to ejaculate. Ejaculation no longer signals the end of love-making, but is just one of the many delightful experiences that are part of sacred sex.

Once you have learnt the basic method for extended sexual pleasure, both women and men can try adding in these Tantric elements:

- Connect with heart chakra of your partner, through your breath and visualization (see page 131)

- While being pleasured, focus on your breathing; remain still, breathing slowly and deeply.

- Focus on drawing your energy up the inner flute (central energy channel) into your heart chakra.

- Visualizing energy moving into your higher chakras: Extend your sexual pleasure by drawing up the pleasure associated with the base chakra into the heart, where it manifests as joy. From there the sexual energy can be drawn into the crown chakra, where it manifests as bliss.

- Try this meditation: As orgasm starts breathe in deeply and slowly, and as you breathe out make as much noise as you can – or sing. According to Tantra teachers, Charles and Caroline Muirs, the volume of your sound influences the volume of your orgasm. They say your orgasm will last as long as you keep vocalizing your breath – as many as several long breaths. As well as that, vocalizing opens your throat chakra, helping pull energy up your inner flute.

  You can imagine pulling the golden sexual energy up with your breath, into your heart, your throat, or your brow centres. Once you have managed to visualize your breath coming up through these successive chakras, you can visualize this golden light streaming all the way up to your crown, and uniting with the energy of your partner. Hold the vision of yourselves as radiant beings surrounded in a rainbow of light, linked to the divine.

- Love muscle squeeze. Experiment with these – men can clench the love muscle if they don't wish to tip into ejaculation. Both men and women can use it to increase the erotic charge in the pelvis.

THE GODDESS SPOT

Robin 37: After going to my first women's Tantra workshop I had a vaginal orgasm with my partner for the first time in 15 years. I've always had great clitoral orgasms, but they're more about tension, having to tense up and feeling more outward. This one was a much fuller, longer experience which I relaxed into. I think that was the reason it happened, I was feeling so much more open, and I felt in touch

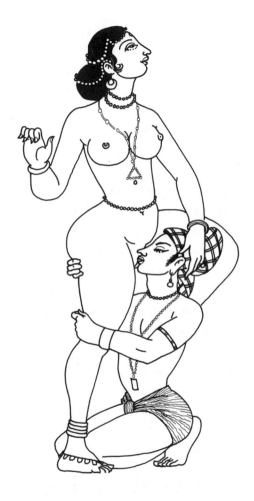

with my own powerful sexuality.

Good sex was always associated with a spiritual connection for me. It had to be very deep and loving. That was because I needed to get love, which wasn't in my life, and I would get tremendously insecure if I didn't feel deeply connected. My need for love meant I would be disappointed. I closed down sexually, because of a lot of rejection and hurt – which I experienced because of the way I'd set it up. I was very hurt by my ex-partner sleeping with other women, and never fully realized it. Now I realize good sex doesn't have to be pure. I can explore a whole range of feelings. I can play with it.

Tantrics call the Grafenberg or G spot the goddess spot, acknowledging its role in bringing women to peak states of arousal. The Goddess spot seems more appropriate than naming it after the man who supposedly 'discovered' this sensitive area of tissue on the top wall of the vagina.

Tantrics describe the G spot and the clitoris as charged sexual poles, one inside and one outside the vagina. Tantrics respect the clitoris as the gateway to sexual pleasure, and learn to arouse it during rituals honouring the yoni. Both the pearl (clitoris) and the goddess spot should be stimulated during extended sexual pleasuring – preferably at the same time.

This exercise is excellent for women who have difficulty achieving orgasm. Although orgasm is not the aim of Tantric sex, it's nice to know you can achieve it before you let go of it as a goal. Orgasm is one of a range of pleasurable experiences you can access during sacred sex.

Women cannot often locate the goddess spot on their own, which is not much bigger than pea-sized. Some women have found it by squatting, and with two fingers inside the vagina, pressing up towards the navel while pressing down above the pubic bone with the other hand (pretty much as the gynaecologist does during an internal examination). It's much easier to find if you're sexually aroused, as the tissue swells and becomes more sensitive. The texture differs from the smoother muscles lining the vagina – it's more rough and bumpy, or ridged.

Otherwise, you can use the yoni massage ritual described earlier to locate the goddess spot.

Stimulation of the goddess spot can lead to female ejaculation, the release of liquid described by Tantrics as divine nectar, the *amrita*. It is light, clear and slightly milky, and it is a Tantric practice to taste it, along with drinking the other fluids of a woman's body.

Exercise

The aim is to locate the G spot and practice combining stimulating G spot, clitoris and nipples to reach and sustain high states of arousal.

The giver needs to be in a receptive state, sensitive to the needs of his partner and giving.

- Find a position in which you're comfortable, where your right hand (if you're right handed) has access to her pearl (clitoris) and your left hand to her vagina. Apply lubricant over the whole area.

- Lightly brush the pubic hair, teasing and gently tweaking flesh. Caress her thighs and the lips of her yoni.

- Circle around the clitoris, gently brushing it with your hand. Stroke the shaft of the clitoris, being careful not to pull back the hood. You can blow over the area, or gently lick.

- Experiment with all sorts of different strokes, changing them gradually rather than rapidly, so your partner has time to relax into the sensations. When your partner is enjoying what you're doing stay with it for several minutes. If she seems to be less aroused, keep your movements gentle until her levels of arousal build up again. She can concentrate on breathing in through her yoni, squeezing her love muscle to draw the sexual energy up into her body.

- Use your thumb at the top of her pearl, while your fingers stroke downwards. Stroke either side, and along the shaft of the clitoris, or circle around it. Keep your stroke slow and steady, at the rate of about one stroke each second.

- A teasing cycle builds arousal. Use a dozen strokes that she finds pleasurable, then do them very lightly for 2 or 3 strokes before going back to the same pressure.

- As she's getting very excited, ask her permission before gently sliding the first or middle finger of your other hand into her vagina. Keep stimulating her pearl in the way that she likes it.

- As she begins the contractions of her orgasm, rhythmically stroke the inside of her vagina. You're trying to stroke her Goddess spot which is in the front and upwards in the vagina – one and a half or two inches inside. Continue the regular one stroke a second cycle you were using on her clitoris.

- When her pelvis contracts in orgasm, lighten your touch, and then switch back to stimulating her pearl. You can maintain her at a high level of arousal and eventually multiple orgasms by alternating between vagina and clitoris, for another quarter or half an hour.

MALE SACRED SPOT;
THE PROSTATE

The prostate corresponds to the goddess spot in women – they come from the same tissue in the foetus. Stimulating a man's prostate produces a deeper, more intense and prolonged orgasm. Alternately stroking the lingam and then the prostate produces a high intensity state of arousal. This sacred spot in men is found by pressing deeply into the perineum (midway between testicles and anus). It can also be reached through the wall of the anus, if your partner prefers. It's somewhere between one to two knuckles in, on the upper anal wall, so you have to curl your finger upwards. You need to be very gentle, and feel around slowly, asking him to let you know how it feels. Like the goddess spot, you can find it more easily if aroused.

The lingam extends a further three inches or so from the base of the penis into the pelvis (towards the anus). The sacred spot is located toward the root of the lingam. Shiva will be able to tell you where it feels pleasurable, and what sort of pressure he enjoys.

It is stimulated to increase arousal. It can also be pressed firmly to turn around the rush for ejaculation, if you wish to prolong love-making.

The aim of this exercise is to build up a high level of arousal, and learn to sustain it rather than tipping over into orgasm with ejaculation. Extending sexual pleasure means that you really experience the full potential of your sexual potency as a reality, realising that it is much more than being able to come as often as possible. Learning to have more control over when and how you reach orgasm means it can become one of a range of erotic possibilities, rather than the be-all and end-all of sex.

Learning to extend sexual pleasure enables you to experience a series of peaks and troughs, allowing you to continue making love for long periods of time in a state of high arousal. You can also experience whole body orgasms, where the exquisite sensations around the penis spread up and through the rest of the body in waves of energy called streamings. These energy orgasms are delightful, and may or may not be accompanied by ejaculation.

- Shiva leans back on comfortable cushions, knees up and legs apart. Find a position where you have good access to your partner's genitals, with your hands and mouth, but where you can maintain eye contact comfortably – usually almost lying between his knees.

- Your left hand will stimulate his penis, and your right hand his testicles, scrotum and prostate, if you're right handed.

- Lubricate his pelvis area and genitals with a good oil or lubricant.

- Touch his penis with a variety of different strokes.

Strokes for the penis:

- Tease the lingam – with breath, feathers, tongue, fingernails, hair, breasts.

- Lightly squeeze, rub and massage.

- Roll the lingam between both hands, as if you're slowly making a fire by rubbing a stick.

- Gently stretch the skin of the lingam from the base up to the head. You can twist the skin slightly.

- Create a ring with your fingers to hold the scrotum.

- Form a ring with your thumb and forefinger of one hand at the base of the lingam, and gently stretch the skin up around the glans with your other.

- Hold the base of the penis with one hand and massage the sensitive frenum (on the underside, where the foreskin joins the glans) with the other.

- Massage the chakra points up and down the penis.

- Play!

After at least a quarter of an hour you can start playing with his scrotum and perineum, the area just behind his testicles, towards his anus. This is called the external prostate or sacred spot:

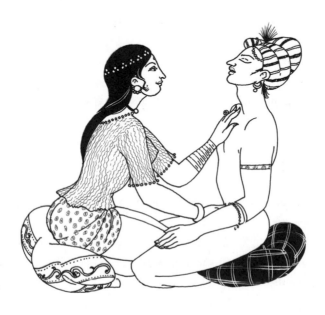

- Steady pressure here feels good, or a firm stroking in rhythm with the strokes you're giving his lingam. You can press your thumb into the sacred spot while hooking your finger around his lingam.

- To build up arousal, you can build up the speed of your rhythmic strokes. He can squeeze his love muscle, and use breathing to build up erotic energy. To slow it down, change and vary the pace and pressure of your strokes.

- You don't want him to ejaculate, so you can gently pull or stretch the testicles if he looks like he's becoming very aroused. Don't stimulate the head of his penis at this stage. Stroke the energy away from the pelvis, especially down his legs, and up to his heart area, as you did during the lingam massage.

- When practising this, focus on not ejaculating. The thin fluid that forms the pre-ejaculate usually signals the start of contractions. Use breathing to disperse energy throughout the body, slowing it right down. Shiva can focus on moving the erotic energy up to the heart area.

- The Taoist, Mantak Chia suggests the man presses down on the PC muscles when approaching orgasm, as though straining to start a bowel movement. Then completely relax those same muscles. Whereas we normally tense our pelvic muscles in building towards orgasm, here we relax them.

- When practising, build up together to high levels of arousal, then come down again, before building up and cooling down several more times. After a while, he'll be able to maintain high levels of arousal without needing to ejaculate, and experience a series of orgasms which are much more like multi-orgasmic women's experiences. He can melt into this state of high arousal, without panting and jerking and preparing for orgasm. He can choose to play with having an orgasm, and with not having one. His lingam becomes extremely sensitive, so a single drop of lubricant, a light blowing breath, or the slightest touch of a tongue can give intense pleasure.

During this experience he draws the blissful sensations from his genitals up through his chakras into his heart, and eventually his crown chakra with breathing techniques, visualization and by squeezing the love muscle.

Part 4:
Divine Sex

'Shakti is always with Shiva.
They are inseparable like fire and heat.
The world is a manifestation of Shakti.'

Swami Sirananda Sarasvati

Relaxing into orgasm

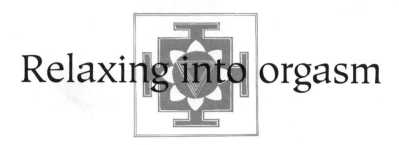

John Hawken, Tantra Teacher: In so-called normal sex, you enjoy what the author Erika Jong calls the zip-less fuck, the quickie, just following your instincts. In some yoga traditions you refrain from ejaculation for the sake of health, purity and higher consciousness and this sets up a conflict between doing and not doing. Tantra refuses to say that you must do this and mustn't do that, Tantra is about being able to enjoy all those possibilities, it's not about being stuck in one way of doing things.

Tantra embraces all possibilities. It's about choice, there isn't one set path you have to follow. This idea is best summed up by the Tantric attitude to ejaculation. The idea is to get in touch with what you really want – what's congruent with your deepest self.

Tantra teaches techniques to draw energy up through the central channels of the body, creating an expanded state of bliss. Usually to build up toward an orgasm, we tense our muscles. In energetic terms, tension involves a contraction inwards, while relaxation involves expansion. It is this sense of contraction that keeps our orgasms focused on the genitals – being more a sense of tension release rather than a sense of expansion. Contraction is also associated with fear, and for many of us with some sort of history of sexual wounding, contraction often feels like the safest thing to do.

Another possibility is to just relax, breathe, soften, and be present to the moment. By doing this, the energy charge that is building sexually can expand rather than contract, literally taking up more space. The energy of the orgasm can spread from the genitals, into the whole body. Tantrics encourage this expansion by visualizing the sexual energy permeating the other energy centres of the body; especially the heart and the crown.

Back to basics – first you need to observe your own build up to orgasm, while self-pleasuring first, and then with your partner.

- There is a moment just when you're about to orgasm, when you feel your muscles are about to contract. To extend this stage, you try to relax into, rather than tense up for, an orgasm. Try to let one or two contractions happen and then relax.

- If you can learn to let one or two waves of orgasmic contractions occur and then relax by breathing slowly and relaxing your abdominal muscles, you can learn to repeat this over and over again.

- Imagine yourself surfing on the edge of a breaking wave of pleasure, rather than plunging over the edge.

- Once you can both do it alone, you can take turns with your partner. One of you pleasures the other right to the edge of the wave, then you swap roles when you feel you're about to orgasm.

- When you and your partner become attuned to one another, you will no longer think about who is on the edge and who is pleasuring; the roles will disappear.

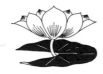

NON-DOING
IN LOVE-MAKING

Leone, 29: I often used to feel that in orgasm mode men are no longer present. I just happen to be there, while he's letting go and depositing this stuff inside me. Then he's gone, he's withdrawn from me and there's a real sense of grief that it's all over. I feel used, and like an object when there's no sense of connection.

Now we're working on making love without any sense of doing, and without orgasms. We start to make love, and then we just stop and lie still with him inside me, just experiencing the sensations without having to go for more excitement, more pleasure.

Non-doing is about letting go of the things I think I want, like excitement. Usually I have a strong impulse to increase excitement, once I feel it. As soon as I do that I'm already goal-oriented.

My fear of not doing anything is that I might lose excitement. So in non-doing I have to trust that something better than the excitement I'm used to, will come along. If I don't just follow my habits, going after what I think I want, I can open myself to a bigger awareness. It's like emptying out, to let something else come in.

In order to experience whole body orgasm, as opposed to a genital orgasm, you need to learn to feel the sensations throughout your body, and to connect your sexual energy with your heart, and with your spirituality. One of the best ways to do this is to give up your attachment to orgasm, in order to allow yourself to fully experience pleasure.

This non-doing style of love-making involves being in contact

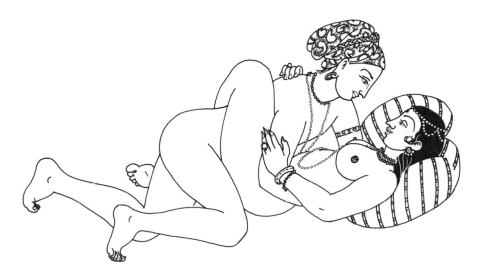

with your partner, deeply connected but without expectations or intent. Just waiting to see what comes into that space you have created.

The art of non-doing in love-making is not to have any particular expectations about what should be happening in love-making, but seeing what arises between you. You both let go of the idea that you have to do anything, that you have to perform. You lie (or sit) with your partner, just feeling their presence, and connecting sexually. Eventually you will find that you don't need to do anything to stay connected with your partner.

One of our tendencies as we get bored with sex is to try to create more excitement through more and more stimulus – doing things in different ways, and trying out kinky activities. Instead of going after more stimulation, Tantra is concerned with allowing more sensitivity, by fully experiencing what's already there. The simple sensation of soft touch on your skin can be extremely powerful.

Whatever you're doing, it's good to maintain eye contact. Keep totally relaxed – it's important not to tense your muscles as you usually do, trying to make something happen. Breathe into your heart chakra, using any of the breathing exercises you feel comfortable with. (For example, synchronized breathing, or alternate breathing.)

You can alternate this total relaxation with squeezing your love muscle, or use a gentle stroking and pleasurable sensation anywhere on the body.

You may or may not choose to have penetration while you're exploring non-doing. If you decide to, penetration is usually soft penetration. The woman can guide the soft lingam into her yoni. This feels particularly nice while sitting in the *yab-yom* posture with spines aligned. By not worrying about whether he has an erection or not, nor worrying about how to sustain his erection, men can let go of their usual performance imperative.

Tantrics believe that the lingam delivers a healing energy just by being inside the yoni, so explore the feeling of the contact between your genitals being gentle and healing, rather than vigorous and exciting. With the lingam inside the yoni in a relaxed way, the positive and negative sexual poles are balanced. The experience of being inside yoni in this quiet, receptive way, is just as healing for the lingam as it is for yoni.

Breasts are also considered women's positive pole; they have a positive energetic charge, like the pearl (clitoris) and lingam. You can stimulate one breast with your mouth while holding the other with the left hand (the hand associated with receiving.)

RIDING THE WAVE OF BLISS

Marek, 45: Before going out in the evening my partner and I did a short ritual. We sat meditating for ten minutes, focusing on the altar, just gazing at the beauty of it. We've found it better if we connect with our own spiritual centre, before connecting with each other. After ten minutes we turned and faced each other, gazing into each other's eyes. We had made an energy circuit, sitting in lotus posture with our fingertips touching the other's wrists, and our left hands giving while the right received energy.

I began to see a different face than her ordinary face. It looked much older, a care-worn, weary face of a woman in her 50s, like a mid European peasant with a scarf on.

We did an Osho meditation, called the *nadha brahma*, under a sheet. We sat facing each other with arms crossed on front of us, holding each other's hands. The meditation is based on Tibetan humming. We hummed to a tape of Tibetan bells in the background, with a sheet over us both.

I could see the candles and the shapes on the altar through the veil of the sheet. I closed my eyes and we played with humming at different pitches, and synchronizing humming and breathing. At first my mind was busy, as usual, wondering whether we should be humming together. Then we found a low note that really seemed to resonate, filling my mind and body, and the space in between us.

We both stopped together after about 20 minutes, and just looked at each other.

She sat on my lap under the sheet. She was wearing a top and short skirt with nothing underneath. I kissed her fore-head, throat and nipples, anointing her chakras with my

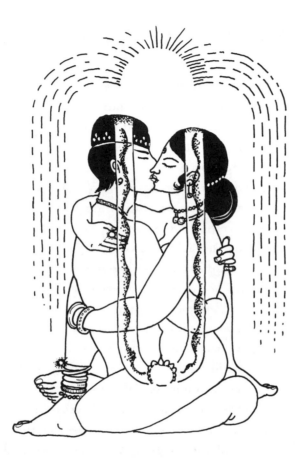

lips rather than oils. I kissed her chakras all the way down her body, then she did the same to me.

We were really turned on, and she sat again on my lap with me inside her, still under the sheet.

We stayed quite still, and naturally started alternate breathing, without moving much.

I imagined a u-shaped tube linking us, with energy sloshing from one side to the other as we breathed in turns. As I breathed in she pulled her hands up my spine, which really helped.

She was getting very excited, even though we weren't moving much. I felt the energy move up through the tube above my head, almost poised there.

What was lovely about it was how equal it was; it was as if we were two halves of the same vessel.

She was really excited, but we didn't go with that excitement. We didn't lose the sense of this magical fluid sloshing back and forth. She reached an orgasm plateau, and I felt very excited but knew I wouldn't actually come. That went on for a long time without any movement. It was unusual staying with not doing.

I didn't get into moving to try and facilitate her orgasm. It was unusual for me just to stay with this equality, not feeling I had to bring her into an orgasm for a peak experience.

We felt as if we were in the same envelope of space – being under the sheet helped that.

Then we separated and sat together holding hands, as we'd done at the beginning. We ended with a namaste, then had a bite to eat and went out.

Ecstasy is not just about peak experiences, although we all like to have these. Ecstasy also has the meaning of *exstasis*, moving away from stasis or stuckness, and into flow. Sacred sex is about entering the flow of energy between the two of you. It's also about uniting the female and male aspects; your inner man and inner woman. This exercise will bring you into the realm of sacred sex:

• After some sexual play of whatever form in which you both get turned on, start this ritual with a namaste bow, then sit in yab-yom position. Get comfortable with plenty of cushions to support you both. The man sits in an open lotus position while the woman sits on his lap, with her legs wrapped around his waist. If she feels too heavy after a while, she can support her weight by staying seated on his lingam, but in a squatting position, which will be easier for her if both of you are slightly raised on cushions. You don't have to start in this position – you can move into it any time that feels right – remember that Shakti chooses the timing, by guiding her partner's lingam inside.

- When your mouths are touching, and Shiva's lingam is inside yoni, a circuit of energy is created. Your joined bodies create a yantra, a mandala of heightened energy which can be circulated around your merged energy bodies without dissipating. You can build higher and higher levels of energy, while areas of the body such as orifices from which energy tends to leak are sealed. The energy you create between you is circulated through your connected energy bodies by means of the breathing and visualization exercises you've been practising in this book.

- At this stage you don't need to join your mouths. With eyes open, gaze at each other. Your heart chakras are in alignment with each other, and you can gaze lovingly at each other easily in this position.

- Start to breathe together. If you're comfortable with alternate breathing go into this straight away. Otherwise keep your breathing synchronized. Keep up a slow, even gentle rhythm. The man follows the woman's pattern of breathing. It doesn't matter whether you both do the female breath (i.e. receiving through the genitals), or the male breath (giving through the genitals, so long as you are both visualizing your energies going in the same direction. Keep up your eye contact.

- Allow your pelvis to rock gently back and forth as you breathe. Tilt your pelvis slightly forward as you breathe inward, backward as you breath out, letting the energy stream from your genitals into those of your partner. This is an extension of synchronized breathing page 142.

- Once you have established the breathing in bringing your hips forward, breathing out, tilting your hips backwards, practise squeezing your love muscle with each inhalation, and relaxing it with every exhalation. With the love muscle squeeze, you are holding the energy you have drawn up into your base chakra, and as you relax the muscle you are releasing it.

- Because there is very little movement to stimulate sexual arousal, you should have developed good control of your love muscle. Visualize the energy coming up into your pelvis, squeezing the love muscle as you breathe in, relaxing it as you breath out and allow the breath to return out through the base of your spine.

- Visualize both your energy as a flame climbing from the base chakra into your pelvis. Pull the energy up with the love muscle, squeezing it to create an energy flow up the Inner flute. You can use the fire meditation here, to help you raise your erotic charge as you draw the energy up through each successive chakra. You should be able to feel energy streaming up your body, from your pelvis, as the sexual charge you are creating between you becomes more and more intense.

- As you reach the top chakra, on the crown of the head, you begin to breathe alternately. When you change to alternate breath you will notice that both your pelvises are now tilting forward at the same time, and backward at the same time – when you breathe out. Still sitting in yab-yom, the woman starts with the inner breath, breathing in through her genitals, and out through her heart, while the man follows the male breath, which is breathing out through his genitals and in through his heart. You can feel the breath of your partner coming out of their mouth. Breathe it in, inhaling their loving energy.

- Now cover your partner's lips with your own, completely sealing the breath. The man inhales through his mouth as the woman exhales through her mouth, still visualizing the inhalation going down into her yoni through his lingam. Then the man exhales as the woman inhales through her mouth, imagining she is drawing his energy from her yoni up and returning it to him through her mouth. This can be done for up to 10–15 minutes, inducing a heady state of oxygen starvation. If it gets too much, just take a breath of fresh air whenever you need to.

- With your mouths together, continue this circular breathing. As your partner exhales, breathe in their warm breath, and imagine it travelling all the way down to your genitals. As you breathe out, send the sexual energy out through your tilted pelvis onto your partners genitals. From there your partner will draw the energy up to their mouth. With your mouths together you become one energy body, circulating energy internally.

- You can then imagine you're circulating the energy through your genitals and your third eye, rather than your mouth. When you're both feeling very aroused and on the verge of orgasm, close your eyes. To seal the energy in your body rather than release it in orgasm, roll your eyes upwards focusing inwards on your third eye, and squeeze your respective love muscles, holding them as you both hold your breath. One of you will be holding your breath in, the other will be holding without any air in their lungs. When it's no longer comfortable, take a breath, and your partner will exhale, and hold. Relax the rest of your body, and just allow the energy to stream upwards through your body.

- Letting go of holding the breath, just allow yourself to breathe naturally, with one partner inhaling as the other exhales, mouths sealing this exchange of energy with sealed lips.

- Now you can circulate the energy right up to your crown chakra, enclosing your whole energy system within one circulating ball of bliss. This feels as if you are part of the complete sexual experience that is life itself.

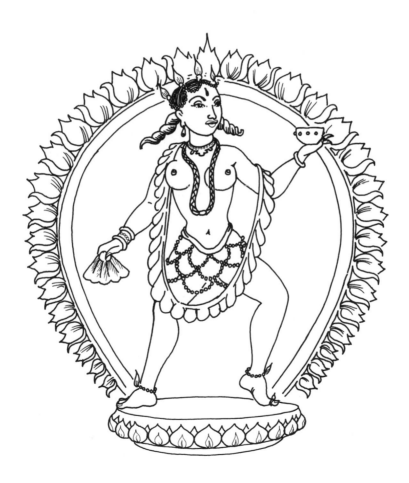

Techniques for mutual absorption include:

• *Exchange of breath, through circulating the breath as in the alternate breathing (see page 144).*

• *The solar lunar breath (see page 130).*

• *Exchange of saliva – through kissing.*

• *Exchange of secretions – through oral sex. The three sacred female secretions are those of the mouth, breasts and yoni. Yoni essence is considered to be sacred fluid. Ejaculate, and menstrual blood are also considered highly charged body fluids – menstruation is considered a potent time for love-making, when the woman should be on top and active.*

• *In intercourse, the man visualizes absorbing female energies through his lingam.*

• *The woman imagines absorbing solar energies through the walls of her yoni.*

Stephen, 28: My partner was a naked goddess, who invited me to sit in her ritual space. It felt both intimate and distancing, like watching a tableau, as she started to dance.

I realised my partner was dancing like the goddess Kali, powerful and even scary. I was trying to protect myself, by focusing on my own internal sense of solidity rather than engaging in the dangerous feeling her dancing created. I felt as if she was waving around a dangerous sword, and that she could maim me. I felt emasculated, but instead of getting defensive I tried to go into receiving mode, just experience what it was like to be in that kind of energy. And of course, that changed the quality of the energy, which became much more erotic.

I was sitting cross legged on the floor, when Leora started to wave her yoni in my face. It felt exciting and erotic, but also I felt honoured that she was showing me her sex like this. Her yoni was in front of my face and she was acknowledging me as a man, and honouring me as her consort. It was like she was coming to me saying 'Here, this is the root of my sexuality. Here it is as a gift'.

I was sitting in the Ganesh mudra, all squinty eyed, with my tongue out. Suddenly she parted her lips with one hand, her yoni was dripping juice and she shook some juice onto my tongue.

I felt it was a beautiful gift.

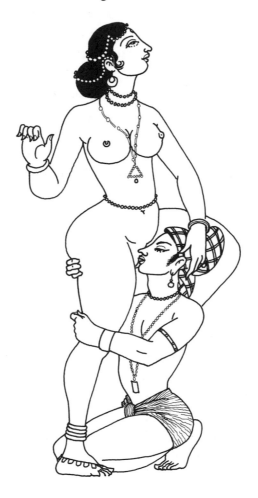

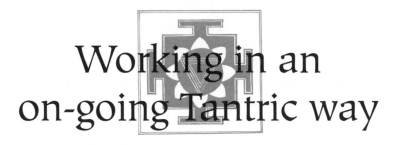

Working in an on-going Tantric way

Bill, 47: Creating a routine for Tantra is important, keeping it a priority and making time regularly. It's about commitment – it's too easy to let other things get in the way. It's important to take time. To spend time stroking each part of your lover's body – getting permission for everything. I ask my lover, 'may I stroke your face,' before doing so. These are the simple things which you miss out on by going straight for sex.

And it's important just to have fun – to have straightforward, good, raunchy sex.

It's important to keep things fresh. What's true for me changes over time. Once I've done something, for instance once I've explored non-doing in sex, my feelings might change and I might want to explore strongly charged sexual energy. You need to explore whatever it is you're both drawn to. If you're drawn to different ways of expressing your love then the yin-yang game is a good way to explore your own needs and desires together with your partner.

Different layers emerge of what feels right for me. Sometimes we flow together easily, and sometimes we go through stages of intense polarization in the relationship. These are usually precursors to moving together to greater harmony.

Communication is vital. We always share our experiences afterwards. We always give each other appreciation – even if things are difficult between us. We appreciate having the space to explore things, however they happen. It's important not to get hung up on a goal. It doesn't help to think about things as having a peak or an end-point – relationships aren't like that.

A sense of the sacred is really missing in most people's lives. For most of us, church or some organized religion is what's on offer. Yet religion may feel irrelevant. Tantra is about finding a sense of the sacred, not out there, but inside. It's about realizing this sacredness in everyday life, and celebrating your existence with joy and love.

Tantra isn't an organized religion, it's a path of the heart. As a path of the heart, it celebrates your relationship with your beloved. By honouring the love you experience with your lover, these feelings can be developed to clear away daily irritations and frustrations between you. Letting go of your self-centred ways of relating to your partner, which stem from an egoistic concern with yourself, and opening up to the grace of the experience of love, enables you to feel this love more and more.

Many couples find they need to do some couples workshops together to help overcome the frustrations and polarizations of their relationship, or to reignite the fire that attracted them to each other in the first place.

As a path of fire, Tantra can sometimes burn because of the intensity of the feelings that are released when you start to work together in this way. This is another reason why it's often helpful to start your Tantric journey with some experienced teachers, who can guide you through the difficult process of not attaching too much importance to some of the strong emotions that can be released through doing exercises together.

Attending workshops helps you to connect with a community of like-minded people, who are working on themselves and their relationships in this way.

A Tantric community can be important to keep in touch with other individuals. Many couples say it's good to practise with other people, in a structured, boundaried way. It's good to connect with other couples to talk about what you're doing. It can also be helpful having a 'buddy' of the same sex, to talk over experiences and what's happening in the relationship. For men it's often a relief to talk to other men about your own sexual experiences – and it can be very helpful to get feedback from someone with a different perspective from your partner.

Workshops are also good for inspiration – to give you ideas about the kinds of things you can take home with you, and integrate into your daily life.

It's easy to follow instructions in a workshop. In workshops, someone is there holding the intention, and creating a sacred space for you. When you practise Tantra at home it's very important to create the right sort of space, so that your connection becomes heartfelt and spiritual as well as sexual.

Use ideas you glean from workshops and from books to enrich your relationship. There are a number in the bibliography which are inspiring to read.

It can be difficult integrating Tantra in your life. Making a commitment to working with Tantra is making a commitment to your relationship. It is a discipline, and like any discipline it needs to be practised to establish it as a habit. Making a regular time commitment is very helpful. Just as you would go to an exercise or dance class every week, you need to make a regular date for your Tantra practice.

A good way to keep the balance in each relationship is for each of you in turn to take responsibility for the session, ensuring that everything runs smoothly.

In a couple you can agree to alternate taking charge of it. You can decide together beforehand what sort of exercises you want to do, or you can leave it up to one of you to guide the other.

The next session that you have together can be led by the other person, so that each of you has a chance to explore your own sexual-spiritual connection.

For love partners it's also good to have time apart – either pleasuring yourself on your own, or spending time with others.

As you can see, there isn't any one style of Tantra, so there's no right way and there's no wrong way of doing it. The exercises suggested in this book are ones to get you going on your own Tantric path. Once you're on your way, you won't need signposts to tell you how you're doing. You'll know from your greater intimacy and your more loving connection with your partner that whatever you're doing is working well for you.

Your body will feel much more alive and you'll be conscious of how your energy moves when you're sexually engaged. Your orgasmic potential will develop into a whole-body sensuality over time, and sexual delight will transport you into realms of bliss you thought were reserved for paradise.

All ecstatics have discovered their own personal paths through the ecstatic process itself. You will receive inspiration and insights as you travel on the journey. Once you're in this realm of sexual magic, you have learnt how to unlock the gateway to other worlds of enchantment and bliss.

Enjoy!

ONGOING TANTRA

John Hawken, Tantra teacher: The path of Tantra goes on and on, endlessly changing. As soon as you arrive at one point it brings up new questions and areas to explore. For instance, once you work on healing shame about your body or past experiences you come up against the question of what's possible. Once you take away the negativity that has been limiting and hampering you, you dissolve into form-lessness and you ask yourself, what is a different form for this energy?

Instead of asking what do I want, how do I get my plea-sure, you ask what do women really want. You ask, what does my partner really want. And then, when you think you've found out, you need to check in with yourself about what you really want yourself.

You discover there are no answers, there is only the journey.

It's like a dialogue between yourself and your beloved of constant discovery.

There's no goal and no set of answers – it's a journey that contains so many questions and answers within itself.

Sylvie, 50: I met my lover in the garden one beautiful spring morning. He challenged me by turning me on in the garden, of course I was embarrassed about the neighbours.

We moved into my Jacuzzi canopy bath. Making love in the water is very healing for me and I love the feeling of floating, and being supported by the water.

We were making love in the bath, and were revelling in the feelings of joy and delight. Usually when I make love my energy shoots straight up from my base chakra to my heart, and if my partner is blocked and can't give, it doesn't work. But my partner's heart was open and we were sharing the joyfulness of our pleasure. Because his heart was open I could receive his sexual energy through my yoni, and I felt my chakras open up one by one. He could also receive my energy and we felt deeply connected. We were in yab-yom in the bath, relaxing in the warm water and looking into each other when my body clicked naturally into this experience that I'd struggled with trying to learn. It wasn't about techniques or breathing in the end, although our bodies were doing that naturally, it was about being open. I could feel the quality of my lover's delight, and the clarity of the energy coming through his penis – without shame and without any holding back at all.

I feel I really learnt for the first time what it means to be open as a woman, and to really receive a man's sexual energy through his lingam. I felt myself opening through his penis. This man opened me up, and I opened myself to him.

I felt my lover's energy course through my body and come out of my head and then back into his body.

I always thought that opening the inner flute would be cathartic, and like an experience of fireworks, but instead it was incredibly gentle and soft, and went on forever. I felt totally peaceful and harmonious, there was no sense of time. I can't describe it, it was like the highest form of meditation I've ever experienced. It felt like a transcendence of my human condition, and a true meeting of my highest essence. It was a quality of expansion I've never had before, and it was gracious.

It's not like a powerful surge of energy, but a streaming of very fine energy without any bars at all. I felt every cell in my body was vibrating at a high frequency, and I'm sure that a transformation must have taken place at some level.

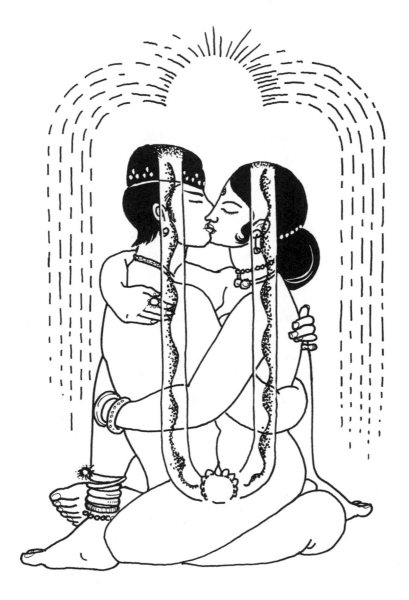

Glossary

Ajna The brow centre is called ajna (command from above), and is represented by two lotus petals connected to a lunar disc, which is positioned to receive the nectar that drips down from the thousand-petalled lotus at the crown of the head.

Amrita The nectar of bliss that rains down on creation from the lovemaking of Shakti and Shiva.

Anahata The heart chakra. This subtle energy is the creative energy of the void.

Bindu Energy point. Usually a dot at the centre of a yantra, which represents the source of energy in the universe.

Brahmin Upper caste Hindu.

Chakra Literally, wheel. It represents a concentration of energy in our subtle body.

Hatha Yoga The word *ha-tha* means sun-moon. In Tantra, hatha yoga is used as a means of preparing the body for more advanced energy work.

Ida The channel associated with solar energy. The current of energy arises on the left side of the base of the central axis, and departs through the right nostril.

Kali The feminine version of kala, time. Kali means time, death and blackness. The goddess Kali is a black goddess who represents the cyclic round of existence, through death and rebirth.

Kaula The word comes from *kula*, meaning ultimate reality, as well as family/group. An esoteric Tantric branch who aspire to the blissful union of Shakti and Shiva, considered by other branches to be left hand practitioners, because of the central role of women, and sacred sex. It was an important early school of Tantra with considerable influence throughout north India. They worshipped the goddess Kubjika, and emphasize Shakti worship in both theory and practice.

Kundalini The serpent power located at the base of the spine, which is our own personal storehouse of shakti energy.

Lingam Phallus. Literally meaning 'mark', the erect phallus symbolizes Shiva consciousness, transcendence.

Maithuna Ritual intercourse. Refers to the traditional ritual practice of making love as the divine, recreating the moment of creation as Shakti and Shiva. It used to take place in a sacred circle, where the central couple made love as the goddess and god, within a circle of initiates who either witnessed the act (without voyeurism) or also participated with their partners.

Mandala Circle. The word had several meanings. It described an outdoor earthen platform used for rituals, as well as a ritual space, a circle of friends, and an assembly. As an enclosed sacred space, mandala also refers to the yoni in Tantric usage.

Mady Alcohol, a substance considered unclean by orthodox Hindus. Tantric rituals can include sharing a glass of wine together.

Mamsa Meat, another food item considered unsuitable for vegetarian Hindus. A shared Tantric meal will include some meat as one of its components.

Matsya Fish. This is included in a Tantric meal because it is generally considered unclean.

Mantra (invocation) Literally a tool to thought. Sacred sounds used to align oneself with the divine. The famous mantra *om* is considered to be the sound of the universe vibrating.

Manipura The third chakra, means to shine like a jewel. It is associated with fire and is located in the solar plexus.

Mudra (gesture) Mudra usually means a ritual gesture in devotional worship, a gesture using the hands which invokes the presence of a deity. It also refers to the toasted kidney beans that are used as an aphrodisiac in Tantric rituals, and in Tantric Buddhism it actually refers to the female partner in couple rituals.

Muladhara (root support) The chakra in the base of the spine. The kundalini Shakti energy lies sleeping here, with her body coiled three and a half times around a lingam. Symbol of the interconnectedness of the Shakti and Shiva principles.

Nadi (current) Energetic channels in the body which have been mapped by Tantric practitioners, in order to know how to move energies around the subtle system of the body to bring about spiritual growth.

Namaste The Hindu form of greeting, where you hold your hands together as if praying. In Tantra it is used to mean 'I honour you as an aspect of myself' or 'I honour you as an aspect of the divine.'

Om This sacred sound is considered to be the sound the universe makes in its natural state of constant vibration. It is used as a mantra to attune oneself with the energy vibrations of the cosmos.

Pingala The current of energy which spirals around the central sushumna channel in the spinal chord, which arises on the right side of the spine and exits thorough the left nostril.

Puja Worship and devotion. Tantrics elevated this aspect of religious worship in India.

Rajas The energetic quality of passion and activity, which all of us have in our character to some degree.

Sattva The energetic quality of lucidity.

Tamas The energetic quality of inertia and darkness.

Sahaja (innate) Refers to the idea that we have a storehouse of kundalini energy which is in-born and in dwelling. Our true nature is always within, we merely need to uncover it.

Sahasrara The crown chakra represents enlightenment – symbolized by the full flowering of the subtle body into the thousand-petalled lotus .

Shushumna The most gracious – the pathway that is the royal road to transcendence. This is the central channel which is rooted at the base of the spine and climbs up along the spinal chord and out the crown of the head, linking the microcosm of the body with the macrocosm of the universe. The central energy channel of the body is called the sushumna, known in Sky Dancing Tantra as the inner flute. Spiralling around the sushumna are the ida and pingala channels.

Shakti The principle of divine goddess energy in which the whole of reality is embedded.

Shakti-Kundalini Universal Shakti energy is found in our own body as kundalini energy, which is thought to lie coiled up at the base of the spine, until awakened through spiritual practices.

Shakti-Shiva The unification of the divine in sacred sex is a primary metaphor for the unification of opposite aspects of the universe, such as immanence (Shakti) and transcendence (Shiva), as well as the female and male poles in us. This metaphor is about becoming whole. The Tantric concept of unity, oneness with the divine is often expressed as Shakti-Shiva, a unification of both energy and consciousness.

Shri Yantra This *yantra* is dedicated to a form of the goddess, Tripura Sundari. The design is made of five downward pointing triangles, which represent Shakti energy, and four upward pointing triangles, which symbolise Shiva energy. Where they intersect they form 43 small triangles, or yonis. This is encircled by 29 mother deities, then another 16. Another circle of 16 lunar energies surrounds these, then 16 lotus petals, symbol of transformation, containing more deities. the central energy point or *bindu*, represents the *shakti* power which is the locus of bliss.

Svadisthana (place of pleasure) The second chakra found in the navel, is associated with creativity, fertility and sexuality.

Tantra Literally means a tool for expansion. As a spiritual path, it has been used for thousands of years as a tool for expanded consciousness, involving expansion on an energetic, psychological and physical level. The word *'tan'* translates as weaving and expansion, *'tra'* means tool. Tantras are literally tools for expansion.

Tattva Essential principle, substance making up reality.

Veda Sacred Hindu text.

Vissudha (purified) In the throat region is the sixth chakra and it is connected with the element ether, the feminine power of creation.

Yantra Yantra is a visual representations of inner and outer energy processes in geometric form. They are used as tools in meditation to help the meditator align herself with appropriate energy flows, and they represent the energies associated with the deity.

Yoni (Vulva) In Hinduism and Tantra the female genitals stand for shakti energy, or immanence. *Yoni* is a Sanskrit word for the vagina that connotes sacred space or sanctum. In Tantra, the Yoni is worshipped with love and respect,

Yoni-lingam A sculptured representation of the lingam (phallus) arising out of a yoni(vulva), which is worshipped in temples all over India.

Yab-yom (mother-father) In the Tibetan tradition this posture of sexual union symbolizes the ego-transcending consciousness of the Tantric practitioner. It refers to the posture for sacred sex in which the woman sits on her partner's lap, in an open lotus position.

Yoga Discipline and union, it is a spiritual path or discipline.

Yogi and *yogini* (the feminine version) Refer to men and women who practise Tantric ritual or other spiritual disciplines.

Bibliography

Further exercises can be found in *The Art of Sexual Ecstasy* by Margo Anand. Thorsons 1999

Tantra; The art of conscious loving by Charles and Caroline Muir. 1989 Mercury House, San Francisco, California.

Geshe Kelsang Gyatso *Guide to Dakini Land*

Vajrayogini *The Highest Yoga Tantra practice of Buddha*

Margot Anand *The Art of Everyday Ecstacy* Piatkus 1998.

Charles Breaux *Journey into Consciousness* Rider 1990

Atmann and Jane Lyle *Sacred Sexuality* Element Books 1995

Daniel Odier *Tantric Quest* Bantam Books 1997

Mantak Chia *The Multi-Orgasmic Man* Thorsons 1997

Georg Fuerstein *Tantra The Path of Ecstasy* Shambala Boston & London 1998

Suyata Saraswati and Boddhi Avinasha *The Jewel in the Lotus* Sunstar Publishing. 1996

Nik Douglas *Sacred Sex*

Agehananda Bharati *Tantric Traditions* Hindustan Publishing Corporation Delhi 1993

Mookherjee and Khanna *The Tantric Way*

Ajit Mookherjee Kali: *The Feminine Force* Destiny Books, Vermont (Thames and Hudson) 1988

Miranda Shaw *Passionate Enlightenment* Princeton University Press 1994

Osho *Tantric Transformation* Element books 1978

Caroline Myss *Anatomy of the Spirit* Bantam Books 1997

Philip Rawson *Tantra; The Indian Cult of Ecstacy*

Swami Sivanananda Radha *Kundalini Yoga in the West* Timeless Books, PO Box 3545. Spokane, WA 99220-3543, USA 1966

Alan Bauer, Donna Bauer and Richard Rhodes *ESO: Extended Sexual Orgasm* Warner Books 1998

Deepak Chopra *The Path to Love* Rider Books 1997

Resources

Contacts list
Organisations for workshops

Skydancing Institute
524 San Anselmo Ave.
Suite 133
San Anselmo
CA 94960
Tel 415 456 7310
website: www.skydancing.com

Skydancing Institute UK
47 Maple Road
Horfield
Bristol
BS7 8RE
Avon
Tel 0117 983 0958

Leora Lightwoman offers workshops for women and couples.
6 Gilling Court
Belsize Grove
London
NW3 4UY

Transcendence
The Tantra Connection
65 North St
Wareham
Dorset
BH20 4AD
website: www.tantra.uk.com

Charles and Caroline Muir run courses and
sell video cassettes
Source School of Tantra
POBox 69-B
Paia, Maui
Hawaii 96779
Tel 808 572 8364

Music to connect sex heart and spirit
Tapes/CDs

Shantiprem *In the Garden of Love*
Verlag Hermann Bauer KG
Kronenstrasse 2
79100 Freiburg

The Art of Sexual Ecstasy by Margo Anand and Steve Halpern
Sound Rx.
P O Box 151439
San Rafael CA 94915
Tel: (415) 453 9800

Music for love muscle excercises (Tantric bonding, from)
Shantiprem *Music for Lovers.*
as above.
Sophia *Return*
Ivory Moon music
22 Rutgers Rd
Wellesley MA 02181

Music from the world of Osho *Yes to the River*
1991 Osho International Foundation
Tao musaic Venloer str 5-7
D 5000 Koln

Music for kundalini shaking:
Transfer Station Blue by Michael Shrieve
1986 Fortuna records
West Germany

Tantra
New World Music Ltd
The Barn, Beeks Green
St Andrews, Beccles
Suffolk
NR34 8NB

Tape of Leora Lightwoman's talk on Tantra at
Alternatives, January 1999
(Includes meditation: uniting heaven and earth)
Price: £7.00
Made payable to: Wrekin Trading
13 Picadilly Mill
Lower Street
Stroud
Gloucester
GL5 2HT

Websites:

tantraworld.com

tantramagazine.com

www.hubcom.com/tantric

www.tantra.com

INDEX

The Art of Sexual Ecstasy

A Lover's Guide to Sacred Sexuality

By Margo Anand

This highly illustrated landmark book on human sexuality describes the sacred love-making techniques of the East in a totally accessible and inspiring way. Margo Anand's liberating practices can immeasurably extend sensual experience for everyone

This book includes a wide range of methods – massage, visualization, breathing, ritual, movement and fantasy – to enhance pleasure and deepen intimacy. Far from being complex and esoteric, these simple and powerful techniques are accessible to anyone who wants to find a gentle and conscious way of discovering a new sexual experience in which physical pleasure becomes a delight of the heart and an ecstasy of the spirit.

Her sexual secrets include how to:

- prolong pleasure by learning to remain aroused while fully relaxed

- expand orgasm to a full body experience

- recover from sexual trauma

- heal a lack of sexual sensation

- have a multiple orgasm for both men and women

- discover innovative positions for versatility and compatibility

- transform sexuality into a truly spiritual experience

Order direct from the publisher by visiting our website www.thorsons.com or calling our 24-hour orderline on 0870 900 2050.